Small Doses Big Results

How Homeopathic Medicine Offers Hope In Chronic Disease

Karl Robinson, MD

ISBN-10: 1493517767
ISBN-13: 9781493517763

To Melissa
whose persistence
and encouragement
made this book happen

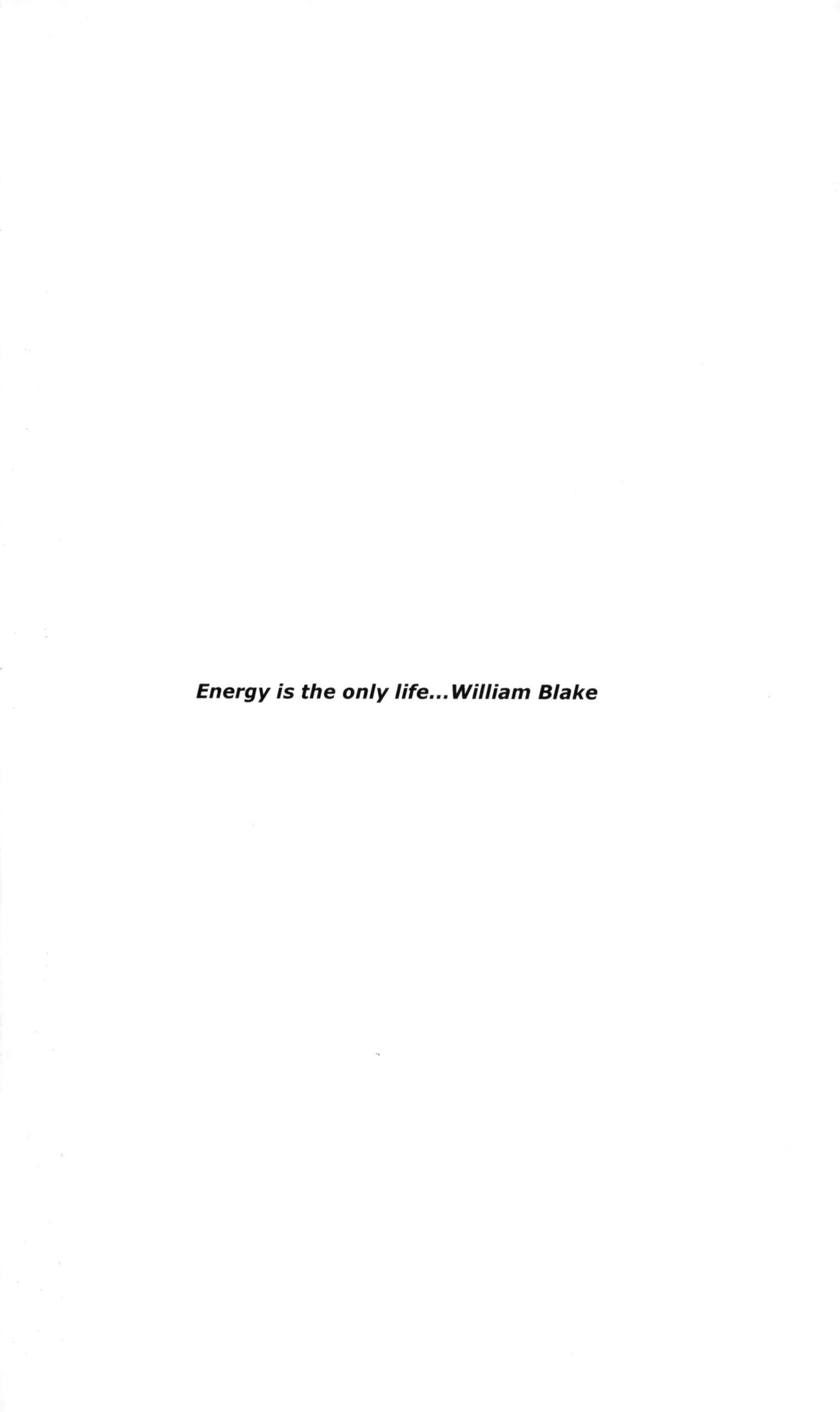

Energy is the only life...William Blake

Table of Contents

Prologue

I came to medicine relatively late in life after a life-changing experience in the Albert Schweitzer Hospital in Lambaréné, Gabon. I was on a world tour in 1966 and 1967, when I injured myself on a motorcycle and suffered a leg burn which became badly infected. I sought help at Schweitzer's hospital which was nearby and was admitted with the diagnosis of "phagedenic ulcer" in which the tissue gets eaten away by bacteria resulting in a crater or ulcer. That was a year after Dr. Schweitzer's death. It was while I was recuperating in the hospital, located on the banks of the Ogooué River, that his daughter, Rhena Eckert-Schweitzer, who was then hospital administrator, brought me several of her father's books and I began to read about his extraordinary life.

Schweitzer was an internationally known theologian, organist, and philosopher who, at age thirty, decided to become a medical doctor and entered the University of Strasburg. Upon completing his medical studies in 1913, he went to Gabon and founded the hospital that bears his name. He spent the rest of his life there caring for the sick.

Schweitzer was a tireless searcher for the truth. One day, while on a lengthy river trip, into his mind flashed the phrase, *Reverence for Life.* He knew instantly that these words perfectly expressed everything he believed in and strove for. More than fifty years later, his words again reverberated, this time in me. Here are a few of Schweitzer's statements that inspired me.

- Ethics is nothing else than reverence for life.
- The purpose of human life is to serve and to show compassion and the will to help others.

- Do something wonderful, people may imitate it.
- I don't know what your destiny will be, but one thing I know: the only ones among you who will be really happy are those who have sought and found how to serve.

Then, one morning, it struck me: **I was to be a doctor**. At first the idea seemed absurd. I was already a successful journalist and loved it. But the idea would not let go of me. I literally could not stop thinking about it. After pondering for the better part of a week, I decided to give it a try with the proviso that if I could not be admitted to medical school within two years, I'd go back to journalism. It was, in some ways, a foolhardy notion. I had carefully eschewed all science courses at Yale except for Geology and Oceanography (every liberal arts major had to take *some* science course). So I had to do all the prerequisites (biology, chemistry, biochemistry and physics) plus sit the MCAT (Medical College Admission Test). Somehow I managed to complete all the requisites in one year and gain admission that same year—a feat considered impossible then as well as now. It usually takes one year to complete the requisites after which one applies. I have always felt it was my destiny to become a doctor and then, a homeopath, so perhaps that explains my good fortune.

I was thirty when I entered Hahnemann Medical College of Philadelphia named after the founder of homeopathy, Samuel Hahnemann. However, when I arrived in the fall of 1968, the only relic of homeopathy was the school's name. It was a thoroughly conventional, medical institution and I duly learned how to diagnose and treat diseases, using powerful pharmaceuticals. I went on to do an internship in internal medicine at St. Vincent's Hospital in Greenwich Village, New York, followed by a residency at Harlem Hospital at 135th Street and Lenox Avenue, New York.

So, why did I, after undergoing an orthodox medical training, turn my back on conventional medicine and take up homeopathy, a form of therapeutics which, in many ways, was a polar opposite to what I had learned?

Call it idealism or an inveterate distrust of the status quo, I became dreadfully disenchanted with the way medicine was practiced. Harlem Hospital, to me, epitomized all that was imperfect about allopathy. Daily, I watched extremely sick people be admitted to the hospital, undergo a variety of tests, receive treatment, and be discharged, only to reappear again two to three weeks later with the same condition or worse, only to receive another round of tests and treatment, be discharged, and so on and on. I saw the disastrous results of adverse drug effects. I never saw a disease, other than a purely infectious one, be cured. I saw a complete disinterest and disregard for the role an unhealthy diet played in causing illness and no interest in how a good diet could promote good health. I never saw my fellow doctors show any interest in the environments in which the patients lived. Of course, the patients were all black and mostly very poor. There was no thought that either the environment or emotional factors could, in any way, contribute to their illness. I saw this enormous disconnect between the mostly shabby conditions the patients were living in on the outside and a coolly detached interest in their deteriorated bodies—their chemistries, urinalyses, x-rays, ultrasounds, cardiograms, etc.

I was particularly dismayed that I was learning to use powerful pharmaceuticals that were often more dangerous to the well-being of the patient than helpful. I did not enter medicine to do harm. All medical graduates are taught, *Primum non nocere,* meaning, *First, do no harm.* This precept, which would appear to be self-evident, is, unfortunately, more ignored than observed. Make no mistake, **conventional medicine is dangerous**. It can be used for great good, but, unfortunately, these medicines carry significant risks. Well over 100,000 patients in U.S. hospitals die every year as a result of drugs prescribed and taken *correctly,* making death by pharmaceuticals the fourth leading cause of death in this country. The number that die from drugs inaccurately prescribed or administered is far higher.

Caveat emptor! (Let the buyer beware!), needs to be applied to modern medicine.

As my disillusionment with modern medicine grew, I began to look for ways to care for the sick that were more effective, gentler, and safe. To my great good fortune, I found homeopathy, a scientific system of therapeutics that, when applied correctly, can be curative for many acute and chronic diseases. What's more, it is safe. For over thirty years I have had the honor and the pleasure of practicing homeopathy. I have traveled the world learning from top homeopaths in India, Ireland, Greece, Germany, Holland, Italy, England, Canada, Argentina and, of course, here in the United States.

It was a great pleasure to work with *Homeopaths Without Borders,* an American based non-profit organization, teaching homeopathy to medical doctors in Cuba.

In the U.S., Melvyn Smith, M.D. and I founded the *Texas Society of Homeopathy,* a forum where people interested in homeopathy could meet and exchange ideas. It holds an annual meeting in the fall that both doctors and lay homeopaths attend.

Later, I began teaching homeopathy in Central America, most notably, in Honduras, El Salvador and Guatemala under my own school, *Homeopathy School of the Americas.* We are now in our twelfth year in El Salvador and Guatemala and over thirty students have become well-versed in the tenets of classical homeopathy.

The interest in homeopathy is rising and will increase as more and more people seek cure rather than palliation and seek to be free of their prescription drugs and enjoy vibrant health.

This book is written to encourage those people who are disillusioned with a system of medicine that manages chronic illness without curing it, who are weary of taking drugs that never cure them, and who wish a gentler, kinder approach to medicine.

–Houston, Texas, 2014

Introduction

There is only one medicine, holistic or otherwise, that treats mind and body **at the same time** with **only one medicine** and does so with **one dose** repeated infrequently. That medicine is homeopathy and, in the hands of an expert prescriber, it is capable of restoring health to those suffering from a wide variety of mental, emotional and physical ailments. It has been doing so for over two hundred years all over the world. Yet, in the United States, it is scarcely known and frequently misunderstood. It has been scurrilously attacked, never by those who practice it, always by those who are certain, theoretically, that it cannot and, therefore, does not work. This book makes no attempt to persuade its detractors and every effort to interest open-minded persons who are weary of being weary, tired of taking pharmaceutical drugs that must be continued, often for a lifetime, and frequently with unpleasant, even harmful, side effects.

I am a duly licensed physician yet my approach to the physical and emotional problems my patients bring varies greatly from the manner in which I was trained. All physicians are taught to take a medical history, do a physical examination, order whatever diagnostic tests are deemed relevant, arrive at a diagnosis, and then prescribe.

This methodology results in diagnosing one or more medical problems with, **almost invariably**, one or more pharmaceuticals being prescribed. That is to say, doctors focus on the patient's **separate** problems located in **various** organs or systems of the body, and prescribe a **different** drug for each problem. Most pharmaceuticals, with the exception of hormone replacements (thyroid, insulin, estrogen, progesterone, testosterone) **force** the body to do something it has no inclination to do. Powerful chemicals drive down blood pressure, manipulate neurotransmitters forcing depression to stay at bay, make pain go away temporarily, etc.

After reading the above to a patient, she said, with alarm, "It's against nature, Doctor Robinson."

For example, if a fifty something patient is diagnosed with hypertension, Type II diabetes, osteoarthritis, migraines, indigestion and constipation i.e., six different medical problems, she will receive six or more pharmaceuticals. As the patient may require two or three medicines to control the blood pressure and two to control the blood sugar, she can easily be taking ten drugs daily, each with the potential of causing harsh adverse effects. Moreover, if any of the pharmaceuticals are stopped, the problem will, in all likelihood, boomerang back. In many cases, the patient is expected to take these meds "till death do us part."

The homeopathic method is the polar opposite. Where conventional doctors focus on separate problems in various organs and prescribe a drug for each problem, homeopaths focus on the organism as a **complete system,** which we treat **as a whole** with one homeopathic medicine. Our idea is to **stimulate a self-healing response** which will **restore order** enabling the entire person to get well. As the physical problems improve, we expect the person to feel better in himself with more energy and a brighter outlook.

Not only can homeopathic medicine be wonderfully effective, it is staggeringly reasonable. Medicine for one month costs only several dollars, and it is included in my consultation fee. By comparison, pharmaceuticals can cost hundreds, even thousands, of dollars.

Homeopathy is a complete system of medicine with its own philosophy of healing and its own medicines which are under the jurisdiction of the Food and Drug Administration in conjunction with *The Homeopathic Pharmacopoeia Convention of the United States.*

The purpose of this book is to explain, as simply as possible, what homeopathy is all about, and to contrast it with the current medical model which I shall refer to as **conventional medicine** or **allopathy** (see Chapter One).

Conventional medicine is expensive, toxic, and often of questionable efficacy. Diagnostic workups can easily cost thousands of dollars. Most pharmaceuticals are exorbitantly costly **and** can cause devastating adverse effects. In chronic disease they are often continued for months and years, never curing, at best maintaining. Even in acute illness (childhood ear infections, for example), one antibiotic resolves one episode for a few weeks. The otitis returns and another round of antibiotics is prescribed, and on and on, throughout the winter.

Homeopathy, besides being universally affordable, is safe, i.e., there are no adverse side effects. And, when prescribed carefully, it can successfully resolve stubborn, chronic illnesses that conventional medicine can only palliate. This book emphasizes homeopathy's effectiveness in the many **chronic** diseases yet includes a number of acute illnesses in which homeopathic medicine played a curative role.

According to the Centers for Disease Control and Prevention (CDC) http://www.cdc.gov/chronicdisease/ seventy percent of all Americans eventually succumb to one or another of the many chronic illnesses.

Chronic disease lasts. It goes on and on, silently undermining health. It is the quiet ravager and it invariably wins. Conventional medicine can throw its many pharmaceuticals at it like so many little Dutch boys sticking finger after finger into the leaky dike but the dike leaks on. Homeopathy, for over two hundred years, has offered a strikingly different paradigm with the possibility of actually restoring health and reducing or eliminating pharmaceutical drugs. It is my earnest wish that more and more people will come to understand, appreciate, and use this wonderful medicine.

Part I deals with the principles and methodology of homeopathy. Part II shows these principles in action with reports of successfully treated patients. Part III explains how homeopathy, unlike allopathy, embraces both the objective nature of disease **and** the subjective, both hard data and the invisible world of sensations and feelings.

Part I

Principles & Practice of Homeopathy

one

Basic Concepts

Much of this book will illustrate homeopathy in action. Cured cases will present various homeopathic concepts and explain how the curative medicine was chosen. But first we have to discuss the basics. Because these principles are mostly unfamiliar, they will be repeated in different ways until, hopefully, you will begin to think like a homeopath.

So, let's begin.

HOMEOPATHY—WHAT SOMETHING CAN CAUSE, IT CAN CURE

The statement, "What something can cause, it can cure," is extreme shorthand for describing homeopathy.

So let's take it in steps. When someone ingests something, be it a chemical compound, a mineral, a plant or an animal product, he or she is very likely, depending on the dosage, to react to that substance and show symptoms. Now, by altering the dose of that same substance and making it smaller, much smaller, it can take away the very symptoms it produced.

To state it another way, if you ingest arsenic, not enough to kill you but enough to sicken you, you are showing symptoms of arsenic intoxication. A homeopathic dose of arsenic can remove those symptoms. (See Chapter Eight for a dramatic example.)

Experiments have been done on mice injected with arsenic trioxide to the point where they suffered liver damage. They were then treated with homeopathic *Arsenicum album* which caused the mice to excrete, via the urine, the arsenic trioxide and the liver damage was reversed.

Other experiments were done in West Bengal, India, and Bangladesh on villagers suffering from arsenic poisoning as a result of drinking contaminated well water. Those villagers treated with *Arsenicum album* compared to those given placebo, showed statistically significant improvement.

The substance ingested does not have to be toxic in order to produce symptoms. Plants not at all toxic can produce symptoms. Salt (sodium chloride) produces symptoms. In fact, microdosages of salt have produced hundreds of symptoms and a homeopathic preparation of salt, *Natrum muriaticum,* is a major homeopathic medicine. Millions of people show unpleasant effects from cow's milk. Those "effects" we homeopaths call "symptoms." Others simply refer to it as "lactose intolerance."

Virtually anything, if given to persons who are **susceptible** to it, can cause symptoms. This is the basis of allergy. A bee can sting one person and kill him, sting another and make him very sick, sting a third with scarcely a reaction. On the other end of the spectrum, there are people with arthritis who deliberately endure bee stings and report they help their arthritis! One man's poison is another man's meat.

Another example is sucrose, table sugar. Most people notice nothing from a teaspoon or two of sugar in their coffee. Eat a pound of sugar a day and you might very well begin to feel sluggish or worse. For those supersensitive to sugar, even a teaspoon will make them ill.

Consider the anesthetics used in surgery. If the anesthesiologist does not inject enough, you will not go unconscious and they dare not begin the surgery. With the correct dosage, coma is induced. A very large dose could kill you.

The same applies to more subtle phenomena. An hour of direct sunlight over the course of a week will cause most Caucasians to gradually tan. Walk for six hours between May and September in the Arizona desert and you stand an excellent chance of dying. Many Latinos die every year walking this desert. If you are very sensitive to the sun, fifteen to twenty minutes will cause a headache.

So foods, chemicals and vibratory phenomena of all sorts can produce symptoms depending on 1) the **susceptibility** of the person, 2) the dosage.

The idea of homeopathy, however, is to use the substance that produces unpleasant effects, convert it into a medicine and use it for curative purposes.

Whatever a substance can cause in the way of symptoms, that same substance in homeopathic doses can take them away.

When Dr. Samuel Hahnemann, the originator of homeopathy, made this observation over two hundred years ago, he stated it as a principle which became known as the **Law of Similars**. "Let Likes Be Treated By Likes," is another way to state it. We also call the most similar medicine the **simillimum**.

MORE EXAMPLES

Think about what happens when someone drinks too much coffee. For one person it may be a sip or two; for another, it's a full pot. Whatever the amount, familiar symptoms will appear. At first, alertness is increased. Later, the mind races, preventing sleep. The nervous system is affected and the person feels on edge and anxious. The heart often speeds up, sometimes skipping beats. According to homeopathy, the best antidote to coffee poisoning is—coffee. However, only a very small amount (one drop or less) will reverse the effects – and then only if that drop is suitably prepared according to exact homeopathic instructions. (Chapter Two)

Homeopaths use two preparations of coffee, *Coffea cruda* and *Coffea tosta,* raw coffee and roasted coffee.

Another example is a cook slicing an onion. Her eyes burn and water profusely; her nose is affected with sneezing and watering. If a person has not been cutting onions but experiences these symptoms, he or she is probably suffering from allergies or the common cold. As one might expect, one remedy for such a condition is *Allium cepa* (Latin for onion) – again a minute amount prepared according to exact homeopathic instructions.

WHERE DOES HOMEOPATHY COME FROM?

Homeopathy is the brainchild of the German physician, Samuel Hahnemann (1755-1843). Although a qualified physician, he was so appalled at the medicine of his day, which was based on a strange theory of "humors" and employed venesection (bleeding patients by opening a vein with a knife) and violent purgatives, that he abandoned medicine and instead made his living translating scientific and medical works from various European languages into German. Hahnemann was a consummate linguist having mastered all the languages of Europe as well as Greek, Latin and Arabic. It was during this period, as he was translating *A Treatise on the Materia Medica* by William Cullen, a Scottish physician, that he read Cullen's claim that the drug, China (other names are Cinchona, Peruvian Bark), was effective in the treatment of intermittent fever (known today as malaria) because it was a bitter astringent and had a tonic effect on the stomach. Hahnemann was acquainted with China and strongly disagreed with Cullen's explanation. In order to find out exactly what the true effects of China were he decided to experiment on himself by taking the drug as it was usually prescribed. Within a period of hours he found himself falling sick with symptoms very like those of intermittent fever. In Hahnemann's own words:

> I took by way of experiment, twice a day, four drachms of good China. My feet, finger ends, etc., at first became cold; I grew languid and drowsy; then my heart began to palpitate, and my pulse grew hard and small; intolerable anxiety, trembling (but without cold rigor), prostration throughout all my limbs then pulsation in my head, redness of my cheeks, thirst, and, in short, all these symptoms, which are ordinarily characteristic of intermittent fever, made their appearance, one after the other, yet without the peculiar chilly, shivering rigor.
> Briefly, even those symptoms which are of regular occurrence and especially characteristic - as the stupidity of mind, the kind of rigidity in all the limbs, but, above all the numb, disagreeable sensation, which seems to have its seat in the periosteum, over every bone in the body - all these make their appearance.

This paroxysm lasted two or three hours each time, and recurred if I repeated this dose, not otherwise; I discontinued it, and was in good health. (Brit. Jour. of Home. Vol. 24, p. 207. Ameke, p. 103.)

Hahnemann, to his astonishment, realized that China had produced, on his previously healthy body, a great many of the symptoms associated with intermittent fever. He wondered: did China cure intermittent fever because it created, as he phrased it, an "artificial antagonistic" symptom complex that resembled intermittent fever? He continued to experiment, not only with China, but with other medicines of his day and, as he did, he became more and more convinced that each medicine could make previously healthy persons sick. Hahnemann called this phenomenon an "artificial disease" as it was caused by the medicine. He experimented on himself, his children and associates. He observed that when a number of experimenters took a given medicine, more symptoms appeared than when only one person took it. All symptoms produced by each medicine were meticulously recorded. These medicinally produced symptoms numbered in the hundreds, sometimes, thousands, and affected the intellect, the emotions and all parts of the body as well as the physiological functions. Each medicine, it seemed, had a global effect on the persons who took it.

Out of these experiments, which continued for years, Hahnemann was able to postulate that that which can produce a set of symptoms in a healthy person can remove those symptoms when they occur in a sick individual.

Eventually, Hahnemann tested his theory in the clinic. When a sick person came in for treatment, he carefully noted all their symptoms and then gave them one of the many medicines he had tested. He chose the medicine that had produced in healthy persons symptoms which most closely corresponded to those of the sick person. To his growing satisfaction, he found that the patients got well. As more and more patients responded curatively to the medicine that most closely mimicked their symptoms, he declared, **Similia similibus curentur**, or, **Let Likes Be Treated by Likes**. Homeopaths refer to this concept simply as **The Law of Similars.**

Hahnemann called his system "homeopathy" with **homeo-** derived from the Greek word, "**Omoios**," meaning **similar** and **-pathy** derived from the Greek word, "**pathos**," meaning disease or suffering. The word, pathology means knowledge of disease and is derived from pathos.

ALLOPATHY

Homeopaths have dubbed regular medicine, **allopathy**, from the Greek prefix, allo- meaning other. It refers to the treatment of disease using medicines that oppose or go against the illness.

Homeopathy is a system of medical treatment that uses medicines that produce symptoms similar to the symptoms produced by the illness.

Thus, allopathic medicines (pharmaceuticals) employ anti-biotics, anti-hypertensives, anti-depressants, anti-spasmodics, anti-convulsants, and so on. Fond of the language of war, allopaths speak of "fighting" various illnesses, e.g., "The war on cancer," etc. They even speak of their therapeutic tools as their **armamentarium** (Latin, *arsenal*).

Homeopathic medicines are the polar opposite. For example, homeopathic *Opium*, prepared from the chemical substance, opium, is known to cause constipation in physiologic doses. Paradoxically, homeopathic *Opium* can relieve constipation when given in a minute dose. All homeopathic medicines, when given to healthy volunteers, produce symptoms which, when they occur in a sick person, can gently remove those symptoms and restore the patient to health. Homeopaths are fond of using the expression, "Like Cures Like" because what our medicines cause, they take away. Homeopathic medicines **cooperate** with the body to induce a self-healing response.

It is clear that the two therapeutic systems have little in common other than they both treat sick people.

THE VITAL FORCE

We are not mere meat. There is a power; Hahnemann named it the Vital Force, that guides the hundreds of billions of enzymatic reactions going on inside the billions of cells. In sickness, it is the Vital Force that is disturbed, or so we homeopathic physicians believe. This vital energy guides the biochemical and physiological processes to work smoothly and harmoniously in health. If the Vital Force itself is disturbed, it disrupts the biochemistry and physiology causing either too much or too little of the many body substances to be produced. Much as a magnet will cause iron filings to line up, so also will the healthy Vital Force encourage the physical body to function in a life enhancing manner.

The Vital Force animates the body. It is subtle. It cannot be seen or smelled, felt or weighed. Yet it is just as necessary to human life as the sun is to all life on planet Earth. Though it is subtle, it is by no means weak. When the Vital Force falls into disharmony, the biochemistry and physiology follow suit and illness results. When the correct homeopathic medicine restores the Vital Force, bringing it into harmony, the sick are restored to health.

UNDERSTANDING THE VITAL FORCE IS ESSENTIAL TO UNDERSTANDING HOMEOPATHY

Homeopaths operate on the premise that the Vital Force is a nonmaterial essence that animates all living organisms. For Hahnemann, all health and all disease depend on the condition of the Vital Force. He maintains, in his most important work, *Organon of Medicine*, paragraph 9, that in health the Vital Force, "rules with unbounded sway, and retains all parts of the organism in admirable, harmonious, vital operation..."

To get an idea of the Vital Force, imagine a three-dimensional duplicate body which is so very fine and light that it can neither be seen nor sensed. Without it, the chemical-physical body would cease all functioning. Indirect evidence for the Vital Force occurs every time a homeopathic medicine (which is immaterial) causes a sudden, dramatic improvement in a sick individual. (See the case below of the teenager with esophageal ulcers.)

In the *Organon of Medicine*, paragraph 10, he writes:

> The material organism, without the vital force, is capable of no sensation, no function, no self preservation; it derives all sensation and performs all the functions of life solely by means of the immaterial being (the vital principle) which animates the material organism in health and disease.

Hahnemann's idea was that when the Vital Force is disrupted then uncomfortable and unwanted sensations appear which we call symptoms. Symptoms, for Hahnemann and all of us who follow his ideas, are signposts or markers giving us valuable clues as to the state of the vital force. We believe that a headache, for example, is happening in two places at the same time.

- It is happening biochemically within the brain.
- It is happening as a disturbance of the vital energy that surrounds and penetrates the head.

Hahnemann puts it this way in *Organon,* paragraph 15:

> The affection of the morbidly deranged, spirit-like dynamis (vital force) that animates our body in the invisible interior, and the totality of the outwardly cognizable symptoms produced by it in the organism and representing the existing malady, constitute a whole.

In other words, when the Vital Force becomes disturbed or "deranged" in the interior of the body it produces symptoms in the body and mind. These symptoms and the disturbance of the Vital Force are one and the same. Whenever a person experiences a pain or abnormal sensation, there is a corresponding disturbance in the Vital Force.

When it comes to curing an illness, homeopaths believe the correct homeopathic medicine acts first and foremost on the disturbed vital energy, putting it into order. As the vital energy returns to order, it, in turn, affects the biochemical processes going on inside the body, returning them to normal and the complaints cease.

RIDDLED WITH ULCERS – UNABLE TO EAT OR DRINK

Let's look at an acute case. It involved a seventeen-year-old boy whose lower esophagus, where it entered the stomach, was riddled with ulcers. He had come down with the flu five or six days earlier—total body aches, fever, the usual flu symptoms. He took the non-steroidal anti-inflammatory (NSAID), ibuprofen, 800 milligrams, the first day and three times that much the next. The third day he developed intense burning pain in the lower chest and stomach. I saw him the evening of the sixth day. He was in pretty bad shape.

"I can't eat or drink," he said. "If I drink even a few drops of water my stomach burns horribly. It's the same with food."

What to do? He needed fluid replacement and could not drink. He needed food and could not eat. He was down sixteen pounds in six days and still losing. He had been to the Emergency Room the day before and received intravenous (IV) saline. They drew blood. All blood chemistries were within normal limits.

He needed pain medication and could not take it by mouth so they gave him an intramuscular (IM) pain injection. The burning kept on and on and was so extreme he was referred to a gastroenterologist who, with an endoscope, looked directly into the lower esophagus and stomach where he observed many ulcers. That occurred earlier in the day I saw him.

He was between a rock and a hard place. Daily trips to the Emergency Room for IV saline and pain injections were impractical and costly. The gastroenterologist said the ulcers could be caused by bacteria, a virus or the ibuprofen. In conventional medicine, the cause is all-important. A virus might be treated with an antiviral, a bacteria with an antibiotic. If the ibuprofen was the culprit, which I suspected, there was nothing to do but watch and wait. But the ball was in my court. I had to find something that could give him quick relief irrespective of the cause.

With homeopathy, the cause is interesting but it is not crucial. We can still prescribe. For us, it is always **the totality of the symptoms** that lead to the *correct prescription.* Especially important are the *symptoms of the man himself.*

I learned that if he moved, even slightly, the burning worsened. Just as important was the fact he was irritable with the pain and irritable around noise. Those latter symptoms, plus the fact that he was sensitive to conventional pharmaceuticals, lead me to prescribe *Nux vomica,* a medicine known for irritability, intolerance to noise as well as over-sensitivity to chemical drugs. He received three or four drops in water, enough to medicate, not enough to cause more burning.

The next morning we spoke. "I am much better," he said, gratefully. "Last night around eleven twenty, I took two large gulps of water.

There was no pain!" Food still bothered him. I suggested drinking some heavy cream. When I called that evening he reported he was even better and had managed the cream nicely. He went on to a full recovery in the next ten days, eating and drinking all the while.

This example shows how the correct homeopathic medicine, by matching the symptoms of the patient to the proving symptoms of the medicine, can have unbelievably rapid results. Note: I did not prescribe for the pathology, i.e., the ulcers. No, I prescribed for HIM. Once his Vital Force was repaired, the *ulcers had to disappear.*

Incidentally, this boy received only one dose of *Nux vomica* 200c (see Chapter Two on the preparation of medicines). That's right. *One, single dose.* It was enough to equilibrate the Vital Force and set the cure in motion.

I have said, and will do so again and again, that our medicines act principally on the *Vital Force* and not on the physical body.

How is that?

It is the way they are prepared. We know they cannot contain any molecules. If they contain no molecules they cannot interact biochemically as do drugs. They contain no molecules because they are diluted so many times that—by calculation—we know there are no molecules remaining.

So, how are homeopathic medicines prepared?

two

Small Doses – How Homeopathic Medicines Are Made

Homeopathic medicines are approved by the Federal Drug Administration (FDA). Hence, they are legal with their preparation and manufacture controlled and supervised by the FDA.

This chapter tells how homeopathic medicines are made. It may seem tedious but it is one of those things one simply has to know about in order to understand homeopathy. So bear with me. I'll make it simple and brief. If this chapter tells you more than you want to know about how homeopathic medicines are made, then skip to Chapter Three directly. If you want to know more, go to the Appendix.

PREPARATION OF HOMEOPATHIC MEDICINES

To make a plant or herb into a homeopathic medicine, the whole plant is cleaned and then placed into a vat filled with 190 proof alcohol (95% alcohol by volume). The plant is left in the alcohol solution for several weeks. During this time chemicals composing the plant are released into the alcohol. After straining the dregs, a colored solution remains that is full of the chemicals from the plant. This colored solution is called a "Mother Tincture."

Drops of a mother tincture can be given to patients, but this is more frequently done by herbalists and seldom by homeopaths who start with the mother tincture and then dilute it.

There are two scales for diluting. One is the decimal scale, abbreviated as an 'x', and the centesimal scale, abbreviated as a 'c'.

The decimal scale = one-tenth; the centesimal scale = one hundredth.

Using the decimal or 'x' scale one takes the mother tincture and puts one drop into a vial. Then nine drops of pure water are added. The vial is then capped or stoppered and the mixture is **successed** which means shaken vigorously either by hand or by machine. At this point we have a one-tenth dilution. A drop of this solution is placed in a second vial and nine drops of water are added. Again, this mixture is successed. We now have a one hundredth dilution. Done a third time, we have a one thousandth dilution, a fourth time a one ten thousandth solution, a fifth time a one one-hundred thousandth solution and done a sixth time we have a solution containing one part in a million.

This procedure is known as a serial dilution. With each dilution there is succussion. **Dilution + Succussion = Potentized substance**.

All homeopathic medicines are potentized. When the centesimal or 'c' scale is used the numbers rapidly become unmanageably large so we use a code. A 6c potentized substance means it has been diluted one to one hundred six times. A 30c = the one to one hundred dilution has been carried out 30 times. A 200c = 200 dilutions. Some homeopathic medicines are diluted a thousand times and more. We refer to a one one-thousandth potency as 1M and a one ten thousandth potency as 10M.

After 23 dilutions, using the decimal scale, it can be calculated that the solution contains no molecules. For those who remember chemistry, we have diluted beyond the negative of "Avogadro's Number" = 6.02 x 10-23.

Knowing, by calculation, that our medicines contain no molecules and observing that they, indeed, do act curatively, we postulate the medicine must be acting in some way other than biochemically. As you now know, we believe this highly diluted and successed medicine acts on the Vital Force bringing it into balance. By restoring the Vital Force to integrity, the physical and mental entity we call the body, simultaneously begins to proceed toward health.

The seventeen-year-old boy with esophageal ulcers received *Nux vomica* 200c. That means one drop of the mother tincture of *Nux vomica* was placed in a glass vial to which was added ninety-nine drops of distilled water and then succussed. This process was repeated two hundred times. Just imagine a huge table with two hundred 2-dram glass vials stretched out in a line. Then imagine the time it took to dilute and succuss each vial. Yes, making homeopathic medicines is labor intensive. Our language is not conducive to speaking or writing such large numbers so 200c is equivalent to the negative logarithm, 10^{-400}.

Just remember, all homeopathic medicines are made by serial dilution and succussion, a process we refer to as potentization. When homeopaths speak of the 'potency' of the medicine, they are referring to the number of times that particular medicine was diluted and succussed. A 30c potency was diluted and succussed thirty times, a 200c potency two hundred times, a 1M potency (m = mil or one thousand) a thousand times.

INFINITELY SMALL, ASTONISHINGLY POWERFUL

Paradoxically, the higher the potency, the stronger the effect of the medicine. I know it sounds self-contradictory to learn that the more dilute a medicine is the stronger it is, but that is what homeopaths have repeatedly observed over the last two centuries. In fact, the higher potencies, 1M, 10M, 50M, CM, should be prescribed only by a skilled practitioner, and then, carefully.

Now that we have discussed the **Law of Similars**, the **Vital Force** and the **preparation of homeopathic medicines**, it is time to talk about what each medicine can do when prescribed for sick people. That will be covered in the next chapter on **Provings**.

three

Provings – What They Are – Why They Matter

How do we know how our homeopathic medicines function? How do we know what each medicine can cure? We know because of **provings**.

So what is a proving? Let's start simply. Say you don't react well to cow's milk. Every time you drink it, you get diarrhea. Whenever you drink milk you "prove" that milk causes diarrhea, at least in you, an otherwise healthy person. You have just done a mini-proving.

In a homeopathic proving, a potentized substance (mentioned in the last chapter) is given to healthy human volunteers until they begin to show symptoms. This potentized substance could have originated from a plant, a mineral, an animal product (milk, venom, etc.), a simple or a compound chemical. It is given to the volunteers, called **provers**. Whatever the provers' experience is attributed to the medicine. Interestingly, these symptoms occur in all parts of the body and also affect the mind.

The symptoms are then recorded by each prover in a notebook. All the symptoms of all the provers tell us what that substance can produce in healthy human volunteers. The proving symptoms, then, comprise the **data bank** of that particular homeopathic medicine.

Usually, the group of provers numbers between ten and thirty, males and females. No one in the proving knows what they are taking except the person in charge, who is called the **master prover**. In a double-blinded study, even the master prover does not know what substance is being proved.

During the course of the proving, which can last up to thirty days or longer, the master prover periodically interviews each prover in order to better understand the symptoms the prover is reporting. He attempts to clarify each symptom. For example, if the prover reports a pain in the left side of the head, he will ask what time of day the headache began and when it left, the precise sensation of the headache (sore, dull, sharp, pressing, bursting, throbbing, etc.) and what made it better or worse (heat, cold, pressure, movement, lying down, etc.) In this way, the master prover makes a symptom more complete. When the provers no longer report new symptoms, the proving concludes.

Then comes the laborious part. All the symptoms that have been recorded from all the provers are assembled and arranged in a prescribed order (mind symptoms, head symptoms, eye, ear, nose and throat symptoms, etc., right down the body to the toes), At this point, there are hundreds, perhaps, thousands, of symptoms—of the mind and of every area of the body.

Over the last two hundred years there have been diverse provings using metals, salts, plants, milk from many mammals including milk from humans, dogs, wolves, skim milk from cows, and others. These provings resulted in many thousands of symptoms. There are also provings from spider and snake venoms. Remember, the provers are **NOT** bitten by the spider or snake. No, they are given the potentized spider or snake venom, usually in a 30c potency which is quite sufficient to produce symptoms in the provers.

Homeopathic provings are never continued to the point where they cause pathological changes in the tissue. This is to say, no homeopathic medicine has been shown to destroy tissue. So we cannot say that a given homeopathic medicine, in its proving, caused an abscess or caused a bunion or a cancer. Yet our *materia medica* is full of pathological symptoms that describe tissue destruction. This is because toxicological reports were included by Hahnemann in his original provings. Toxicology is the study of the adverse effects of chemical, physical or biological agents on living organisms. Hahnemann, in his provings, included the symptoms of persons who had inadvertently been exposed to a poisonous plant or metal or who were bitten by a poisonous creature and then became sick. Hahnemann was careful to annotate which symptoms came from toxicological reports and which were proving symptoms. Over the last two hundred years, when a homeopathic medicine was found to cure a pathological condition, and to do so repeatedly, it was included in our literature.

Our *materia medicas,* then, are composed of symptoms from:

1. Provings conducted on healthy human volunteers, male and female.
2. Toxicological reports from the medical literature.
3. Clinical reports of verified cures.

To get a slight idea of the diversity of symptoms from a single proving, let us look at the original proving of *Alumina* (oxide of aluminum) by Hahnemann. There were eleven provers including Hahnemann himself. Altogether, they reported 1,161 different symptoms! A tiny sampling follows:

- She cannot see blood or a knife without horrible thoughts pressing in upon her, as if she should commit suicide though she has the greatest horror of it.
- A numb feeling in the head as if his consciousness was outside of his body; when he says anything, he feels as if another person had said it; and when he sees anything, as if another person had seen it, or as if he could transfer himself into another, and only then could see.
- Vertigo even to falling, the whole room turns with her; she has to sit down at once.
- Unbearable itching on the head; he has to scratch until it bleeds.
- Itching burning in the anus.
- Frequent sneezing.
- The nose is stopped up.
- Pain as from a sprain in the shoulder-joint, especially on raising up the arms.
- During the siesta, when he is about to go to sleep while sitting, a jerk through head and limbs, like an electric shock, with stupefaction.
- She talked aloud in her sleep, laughed and wept.

- Pain in the back, as if a red hot iron was thrust through the lowest vertebra.

These few proving symptoms of *Alumina* are amazingly detailed and show how the medicine affected both the minds and bodies of the eleven provers. And remember, these are just eleven symptoms out of 1,161!

That last proving symptom mentioned, pain in the back "as if a red hot iron," enabled me to give relief to a fifty-year-old woman with severe back pain. It was 2002 and the pain was so unbearable that she was taking the narcotic, hydrocodone, daily and going to her chiropractor two to three times a week. Still, the pain was persisting. Frankly, I hadn't a clue what to give her until she said, "It feels like a burning rod going up my spine. It starts in my lower spine and goes straight up." She also mentioned that both her hands had become "numb." Moreover, she said she had a pain from the elbows to the wrists or from the wrists to the third and fourth fingers, "like an electric shock."

Now, this was no ordinary description of pain. Most people say something like, "Doc. I've got this bad back pain. It really hurts. It goes up my back." That's it. They simply cannot tell you more. Question them as long as you like, that's it. So when someone likens her pain to a rod going up the spine and not just any rod but a "burning rod" that is important to a homeopath. But why, you ask, is it important? For one thing, the description of pain is graphic. One can easily imagine a burning rod thrusting up one's spine. But there's another point. A prover (remember, a prover is healthy when he starts the proving) sometime between 1828 and 1836, as a result of taking oxide of aluminum, developed, "Pain in the back, as if a red hot iron was thrust through the lowest vertebrae." So, over one hundred eighty years later, when my patient described her pain in those words, I experienced a "Bingo!" moment. She almost certainly needed a dose of *Alumina.* But I needed confirmation. She mentioned numbness of the hands. And she said she had pains from the elbows to the wrists "like an electric shock." Both symptoms I was able to find in the proving of *Alumina.* She received *Alumina* and slowly over the next two weeks the pain and numbness diminished and went away.

Can you think of any drug used today that has been in continuous use for that amount of time? I cannot. Most drugs today are popular for ten to twenty years then become relegated to the dustbin of disused pharmaceuticals. There is always a newer, "better" drug in the pipeline. It is telling that most of the homeopathic medicines have been in continuous use for nearly two hundred years, some longer.

Understand that all proving symptoms are reported in the words of the prover and contain no medical terms. It is our good fortune that medical terms were not used two hundred years ago, when many of the provings were done, since no one today would understand them.

Realize that all homeopathic provings are done with human subjects. It is very different from the testing a new pharmaceutical drug undergoes. It is tested first on animals and later on patients with a specific disease. Since animals don't talk there can be no information about what sensations the drug might produce or what mood changes might occur. When the drug is finally tested on patients the investigators are mainly concerned with how it affects a given disease. For example, does the new antihypertensive lower blood pressure? Does the antidepressant improve the mood? And so on.

A good homeopathic proving will produce up to two thousand symptoms and will affect many, many areas of the body and mind. So detailed are the symptoms of a good proving that homeopaths often refer to a proving as though it were a person. We talk among ourselves of a *Sulphur* type, a *Phosphorus* type, a *Pulsatilla* type, etc. We speak of these medicines as if they were living people! We'll say, "He's a real *Sulphur*," or "She really acts like *Pulsatilla*." It is homeopathic "code" that refers to the proving symptoms of that medicine which were so detailed that they suggested the way a person who might need that medicine would behave both emotionally and physically.

THE PROVINGS FORM OUR DATA BASE

A homeopathic proving constitutes the data base of that substance. It is detailed evidence of what that substance causes in healthy humans. We consult this data base or proving to find out what the medicine produced in the way of symptoms.

Now here's the interesting part: homeopaths know that ANYTHING A MEDICINE CAN CAUSE IN THE WAY OF SYMPTOMS, THAT SAME MEDICINE CAN REMOVE THOSE SYMPTOMS. Remember—anything a homeopathic medicine can cause, it can cure. This is another way of saying, **"Like Cures Like."**

We consult the proving of a given medicine, looking to see if the symptoms it contains MATCH the symptoms of our patient. When we are satisfied that most of the patient's key symptoms CORRESPOND closely to the proving symptoms, we then prescribe that homeopathic medicine. When we have chosen wisely, the patient returns to health.

It sounds easy, but it is far from easy. Of the several hundred homeopathic medicines in common use, many symptoms from many different medicines are either the same or similar. There is tremendous overlap. So we have to use our judgment, our intuition and our experience to select the most homeopathic medicine, i.e., the medicine that most corresponds to the symptoms of the patient.

Now that the principles of homeopathic medicines have been introduced, it is time to talk about symptoms and diagnoses.

four

Symptoms, Diagnosis and Treatment

SYMPTOMS

There are many aspects of homeopathy that differ from conventional medicine. One of them is how we understand and make use of symptoms. A symptom, generally speaking, is something undesired, either an unwanted sensation (pain, numbness, tingling, fullness, heaviness, etc.) or an unwanted change in the way the body functions (loss of memory, impotence, constipation or diarrhea, urinary frequency, etc.) and is often associated with a disease. Both conventional medicine and homeopathic medicine would agree on this definition.

DIAGNOSIS

For the conventional doctor, a certain configuration of **common** symptoms leads to a diagnosis. Some simple examples:

- **Asthma** is characterized by wheezing respiration brought on by exposure to cold or allergens accompanied by shortness of breath and weakness. The airways, notably the bronchi, become constricted and narrowed and it is difficult for the air to pass.
- **Hepatitis**, an inflammation of the liver, caused by viruses, alcohol, medicines and various poisons, makes itself known by fatigue, fever, jaundice, swelling of the liver, darkened urine, loss of appetite and nausea.

- A **migraine** headache is more severe than an average headache and usually affects only one side of the head. It is accompanied by nausea, sometimes vomiting, extreme sensitivity to noise and light, and there can be visual disturbances.

Note again how the allopathic diagnosis rests on **common** or expected symptoms that, taken together, signify a given illness.

For the homeopath, a diagnosis (asthma, hepatitis, migraine, etc.) is just the beginning of the case assessment. The homeopath wants to know what distinguishes one case of, say, asthma, from other cases of asthma. To do so, we look to what is strange or unexpected or not easily explained in terms of physiology. For example, the patient may say, "Doc, funny thing, but with this asthma, when I get off a good burp, my breathing eases." Two homeopathic medicines have this strange symptom and thereby either could become the medicine the patient needs. I say "could become" because the medicine selected must reflect many aspects, not only of the disease but of the person himself.

Perhaps the asthma came on shortly after a nasty skin condition was treated with steroids, either in the form of a cream or by mouth. In the repertory I use (RADAR), there are seventeen homeopathic medicines known to treat asthma that comes on after a skin lesion has been suppressed. Any one of those seventeen medicines could figure in the final prescription.

Note that the homeopath searches for the anomaly in each case, i.e., that which deviates from what is standard, normal, or expected. We call such symptoms **strange, rare and peculiar**. Symptoms which are common to the disease almost never aid the homeopath in finding the correct medicine, whereas the strange, rare, and peculiar ones invariably do. Ironically, the conventional doctor has no way of taking into account strange, rare, and peculiar symptoms, and usually dismisses them. He holds fast with the common symptoms (see above) to reach a diagnosis.

Let's take another example. A patient has hepatitis A. In the course of taking the case, we find that a week or so before coming down with hepatitis he was humiliated by his boss in front of his colleagues causing him great chagrin. In the repertory, there is one medicine under the rubric, "Abdomen, inflammation of the liver after mortification," and that medicine is *Lycopodium*. Whether or not *Lycopodium* will be selected depends, as mentioned above, on whether the rest of the symptoms point to *Lycopodium.* However, you may ask yourself, "If hepatitis A is known to be caused by a virus, what does it matter if the person was humiliated? It is obvious that the virus was responsible."

Not so fast. Yes, hepatitis A is "caused" by a virus. There is no disagreement there. But the humiliation the man suffered in front of his colleagues was a huge shock not only to his mind, but also weakened his immune system allowing the virus to begin multiplying and damaging the liver. The human body is like a huge and very intricate mobile. Set one part in motion and all the rest of the mobile begins to move. So, yes, the mortification he experienced could have set the stage for his hepatitis.

I have had parallel experiences with migraines. I have successfully treated hundreds of patients with migraine headaches. It still surprises me how many migraines came on after a great grief, the loss of a loved one, the breakup of a relationship, the loss of a job, etc.

TREATMENT

In allopathic medicine the **common symptoms** plus appropriate laboratory tests lead to a diagnosis. The diagnosis dictates the treatment and the treatment is usually quite standard, i.e., there is little debate or discussion. For example, with hypertension everyone receives an antihypertensive drug. With migraines, everyone receives a pain medicine. With bacterial cystitis, everyone receives an antibiotic.

A homeopath has no trouble arriving at the same diagnosis. Strangely though, homeopathic treatment is *not* standardized. Anything but. Five patients with infectious hepatitis could easily receive five different homeopathic medicines. Ten patients with migraines might be prescribed ten different homeopathic medicines.

A HOMEOPATHIC MEDICINE IS NOT *STANDARDIZED* TO THE DISEASE, BUT *INDIVIDUALIZED* TO THE PATIENT WITH THE DISEASE

This is a RADICAL concept and it needs explaining. First of all, a homeopath takes a far more detailed history than an allopath. The diagnosis, on which both the allopath and the homeopath agree, is the endpoint for the allopath for with the diagnosis in hand, the treatment is fairly standard and routine, as mentioned above.

However, for the homeopath, the same diagnosis in no way helps him to prescribe. He continues taking the case in search of minute details that will distinguish one patient from another AND help him to select the medicine most homeopathic (similar) to BOTH the patient and his disease.

The kinds of clues the homeopath is looking for include but are not limited to the following:

- Is the pain localized or does it extend from one point to another?
- Can the patient describe the pain (bursting, pressing, sharp, aching, dull, heavy, burning)?
- What makes the pain better or worse? For example, is a knee pain better at rest or in motion, from applying a hot pack or a cold pack?
- Is the patient affected by any sort of climate or weather?
- Is the pain more severe lying on the right side or the left side or the back?
- Is the pain worse at night or during the day?
- Is there a specific hour during which the complaints are significantly worse?
- Is the patient thirsty or thirstless?
- With the illness does the patient ask for certain foods or beverages or has he become averse to certain foods and beverages?
- How is the patient affected by hot vs. cold temperatures?
- Has the patient's disposition altered during the illness? For example, has he become indifferent, irritable, anxious, fearful, or unwilling to answer?

As you can see, these bits of data often have little to do with the disease itself and more to do with how the patient is REACTING to the disease. As the homeopath learns more and more about his patient, he is constantly thinking, "Now, does he need medicine A or B or possibly C or D? Which medicine best corresponds both to the disease symptoms and to the patient?"

THE DIAGNOSIS IS THE MEDICINE

The homeopath, during the case taking and analysis, is constantly differentiating one homeopathic medicine from another. In this sense, **the medicine selected IS the diagnosis**. By eliminating first this medicine, then that one, then another, he finally decides on one single medicine that most closely MATCHES the symptoms of his patient. His conclusion or diagnosis is: "She needs *Sulphur*," or whatever medicine he decides on.

Let's look at some simple examples. Say we had five persons, each with infectious hepatitis (Hepatitis A). The allopath, having arrived at the diagnosis, would advise bed rest and little else as he has no treatment for hepatitis A. The homeopath has very effective treatments. After taking an extensive history, he might prescribe different homeopathic medicines, depending on what he found.

- A *Phosphorus* patient will be chilly, crave cold drinks, be unable to lie on his left side, and become fearful if left alone.
- An *Arsenicum* album patient will be chilly, intensely anxious and restless (especially from 1 to 3 a.m.), want to frequently sip cool drinks and have a strong fear that he will die.
- A *Nux vomica* patient will be chilly and stay well-covered as the least draft will be unbearable. If asked a question, he will become very irritable. He usually is impatient, and sensitive to noise and light.
- A *Pulsatilla* patient will be overly warm, want cool air, be weepy and desire love and reassurance. She is usually thirstless.
- A *Bryonia* patient will be hot, lie very still as the least movement will cause intense liver pain, and be thirsty. He will become irritable if disturbed.

Remember, all five of these patients have the typical symptoms and elevated liver enzymes characteristic of infectious hepatitis. The diagnosis is correct and both the homeopath and the allopath agree on that score. But the homeopath looks further into each case and learns how each person's reaction to the disease differs from the others. Three of the patients are chilly, while two are hot. One is thirsty, while another is thirstless. Some are irritable. Others are anxious or fearful. The homeopath then DIFFERENTIATES one homeopathic medicine from another. The correct medicine will shorten the course of the hepatitis. Note also, there is no ONE medicine in homeopathy for hepatitis A, not in homeopathy. Each case has to be studied on its own merits and INDIVIDUALIZED. That is a term we homeopaths use a lot. No matter what the complaint, we treat each patient as a unique individual. It's a bit like having a suit tailor-made. Our idea is that the medicine fits the patient just as elegantly and snugly as a new tailor-made suit.

Homeopathy should be making more and more sense. In the next chapter, we'll explore one of our most valuable tools, the repertory.

five

The Repertory

Throughout the nineteenth century, beginning with Hahnemann and continuing with his followers, more and more medicines underwent provings (Chapter 3). These provings, taken as a whole, constitute our *materia medica,* a Latin term that refers to the collected knowledge about the therapeutic properties of all homeopathic medicines. Because some provings produced one to two thousand symptoms, the *materia medica* soon became unwieldy and difficult to access.

All this changed with C.M.F. Bœnninghausen (1785 - 1864). Bœnninghausen was a Baron by birth, a lawyer by profession, and a botanist and agriculturist by way of interest. In 1827, he developed tuberculosis, got no relief from orthodox treatment, and his physicians gave him no hope of recovery.

Believing he was not long for the world, he wrote a letter to his friend, Dr. A. Weihe, with whom he shared botanical interests. He told him of his condition and bid him goodbye. Dr. Weihe was one of the early homeopaths though Bœnninghausen did not know that at the time. Weihe wrote back suggesting Bœnninghausen try homeopathy. Bœnninghausen sent Weihe his symptoms; Weihe analyzed them, and sent him the homeopathic medicine, *Pulsatilla,* by return post. Within a few months Bœnninghausen made a complete recovery and became a firm adherent of this new science.

Though not himself a doctor, Bœnninghausen plunged into an intense study of homeopathy. Because of his training as a lawyer and botanist, he had a keen, analytical mind and soon became an outstanding prescriber. His fame grew, and in July, 1843, King Wilhelm

IV conferred on Bœnninghausen the official status of a practicing physician.

Over the years Bœnninghausen became a close friend and collaborator with Hahnemann who asked him to arrange the thousands of proving symptoms in such a way that they could be easily accessed. Thus was born the first repertory, *Repertory of Anti-Psoric Medicines* by Bœnninghausen in 1832. It was followed by the repertory that made him famous and is still in wide use today, the *Therapeutic Pocket Book*, which was first printed in 1846.

What Bœnninghausen, and others who created their own repertories, did was to take key symptoms from the provings and arrange them alphabetically. Each key symptom was followed by the medicines known to cause (and therefore remove) that symptom.

Repertories vary in the way they are structured but basically one can look up "Anger" and find a certain number of medicines known to cause and cure anger. The symptom, "Chill" will be followed by medicines that cause and cure a chill. The same is true for "Tingling," "Worse cold," Worse heat," and "Worse motion," and "Head pain" and so on and so forth. In other words, there are thousands and thousands of symptoms with many more thousands of medicines following each symptom.

RUBRIC – THE DEFINITION

Homeopaths, by convention, refer to any symptom that appears in a repertory as a **rubric**. So when we use the word "rubric," that is "homeospeak" for a symptom that appears in a repertory.

OTHER REPERTORIES

In the late nineteenth century, the homeopath, James Tyler Kent, M.D., created his own repertory. The layout is quite different from Bœnninghausen's *Therapeutic Pocket Book*, but the idea is the same, i.e., to enable the practicing homeopath to quickly and easily access the many thousands of symptoms in the provings. One can say that a repertory is a kind of dictionary or concordance.

Let's say I have a patient with a tremendous fear of dying. Using Kent's repertory I would turn to the "Mind" section, then to "Fear" and finally to "Death, fear of." and there I would find those homeopathic medicines known to cause a fear of death in certain provers and remove the fear of death in patients. A homeopath never prescribes on a single symptom, however. So let's look at a hypothetical patient.

A patient has asthma. In the course of the interview, one learns he has a bad attack every night at 2 a.m. and jumps out of bed, heads for the frig and sips cold water. He has an enormous fear of death which is worse during the attack at 2 a.m. He is also a very careful, even fastidious, person in his habits.

One can look up each of these symptoms in Kent's repertory and the one medicine that runs through all the rubrics is *Arsenicum album* (white arsenic).

Unfortunately, in real life, it is rare that one medicine will stand out so clearly. So repertories are used as guides. Say a repertorization suggests three or four medicines. We then further quiz the patient to see which of the four seems most similar to his symptoms and we also consult one or more *materia medicas* to read what other homeopaths have written about the four medicines we are considering.

Oh, by the way, in the hypothetical above in which *Arsenicum album* was the correct medicine, before you become alarmed, thinking homeopaths give poisons, refer back to Chapter 2 for a refresher on how homeopathic medicines are formulated. Remember each medicine is diluted to the point at which **no molecules** remain. As Paracelsus is reported to have said, "The dose makes the poison, " or in Latin "*Sola dosis facit venenum*".

Kent's repertory was published in 1897. It has been added to and updated in the last thirty years by modern homeopaths and there now appear two well-known versions, *Synthesis Repertory*, edited by Frederik Schroyens, M.D., and the *Complete Repertory* by Roger van Zandvoort.

Both are in wide use worldwide and both have been made available in software editions. The software program I use is called RADAR and contains the repertory, *Synthesis*. Another excellent software program is MacRepertory which contains the *Complete Repertory*.

THE REPERTORY AS A TOOL

Most modern homeopaths use repertories and most no longer use them in book form but rather as computer software. The advantage of a repertory is that one can swiftly look up a number of rubrics and drag them into a clipboard. The software will then instantly analyze all the medicines that appear in all the rubrics and let one see which medicine best covers the symptoms entered. It will also let you see which medicine appeared in second place, third place, and so on.

Of course, it is not all that simple. The homeopath has to select carefully which rubrics to use and when those rubrics are analyzed, he must further decide which of the first ten or fifteen medicines that appears is the most likely to cover the case. He may then refer to one of several *materia medicas* to read further on each medicine. Homeopathy, correctly practiced, is time-intensive and demands careful thought.

The next chapter will show how pharmaceuticals differ from homeopathic medicines. The contrast is sharp.

six

Medicine Looking For Disease Versus Medicine Looking For Itself

In conventional medicine, pharmaceuticals are molecules created to do a very specific job, which is to cure or alleviate a specific disease or condition. Some are targeted to interact with receptors on the surface of cells blocking the physiological function of a certain protein. Others are enzyme inhibitors, molecules that bind to enzymes and decrease their activity. The point is that modern pharmaceuticals have an extremely narrow biochemical focus. Some examples: there is a class of drugs known as beta blockers that diminish the effect of epinephrine (adrenaline) and is used in the management of cardiac arrhythmias, hypertension, angina and heart failure.

Another class is the non-steroidal anti-inflammatory drugs (NSAIDs). This group of drugs includes aspirin, ibuprofen (Advil, Motrin, Nuprin) and naproxen (Aleve). They block specific enzymes known as Cox-1 and Cox-2, responsible for making prostaglandins, chemicals that cause damaged tissues to swell. NSAIDs stop the body from making too many prostaglandins, thereby reducing swelling and pain.

A third class of drugs is antibiotics designed to kill various types of bacteria. Of course, there are thousands of drugs and virtually all have a chemical action that can be assayed, i.e., tested and measured.

In general, one can say that drugs are created to treat something specific whether it be a given organ, system of the body, bacteria, virus or fungus. In this sense, pharmaceuticals are **medicines looking for disease.**

The same cannot be said about homeopathic medicines. They certainly cannot be assayed. After all, there is "nothing there." Our medicines do not target physical structures. They do not look for receptors or enzymes or bacteria or viruses or fungi. Nor do they target any particular biochemical process or physiological function. **Yet they affect all of these things**. It was Hahnemann's contention that the Vital Force "rules with unbounded sway, and retains all the parts of the organism in admirable, harmonious, vital operation..." (*Organon* paragraph 9)

Homeopathic medicines interact with the Vital Force itself, repairing it, balancing it, and enabling it to exert a benevolent effect over the entire organism. So powerful is the Vital Force that when it is attuned it brings the physical organism with all its biochemistry and physiology into healthy operation. The result is good health.

Of course, the contrary must be true. When the Vital Force is disturbed, it **produces** symptoms as the body falls into illness. The correct homeopathic medicine restores the Vital Force, which, in turn, restores the physical, chemical body to health.

A HOMEOPATHIC MEDICINE IS LOOKING FOR ITSELF

After being serially diluted and succussed, (Chapter Two), a homeopathic medicine has its own unique vibration. When given to a sick person, it resonates with the disturbed Vital Force of that person and brings it into order.

The selection of the homeopathic medicine is *all important* and is accomplished by *following the symptoms.* For the homeopath, all symptoms are interesting in themselves but also as an indication of the deranged Vital Force. The deranged Vital Force produces symptoms so, ipso facto, we follow the symptoms in order to find a homeopathic medicine that most closely, in its proving symptoms, resembles the symptoms of the patient.

Modern medicine is often criticized as doing nothing more than "treating the symptoms." It is a valid criticism. Give pain medicine for a headache and the headache becomes bearable. Of course, the tendency to headache has not been addressed. Homeopathy is **not** treating the symptoms but **using the symptoms as signposts to understand and treat the disturbed Vital force.** By treating and restoring the vital energy it is possible to cure, i.e., restore health, on a lasting basis.

The homeopathic medicine, in its resonating essence, is looking to find itself in the resonating essence of the sick person as expressed by the patient's symptoms

Let's look at one famous homeopathic medicine, *Belladonna.* In its pathogenesis (proving) *Belladonna* mimics inflammation. The medical definition of inflammation is *calor* (heat), *dolor* (pain), *rubor* (redness) and *tumor* (swelling) to which a fifth has been added *functio laesa* (loss of function). Patients who need *Belladonna* often have, running like a red thread through their complaints, the cardinal symptoms of inflammation.

Now, and this is the interesting part: we shall find that red thread in all the following conditions:

1. A severe headache with the head feeling hot, throbbing in the temples, with a feeling of fullness in the head and pain.
2. A sore throat with red, swollen, pulsating tonsils which feel hot, making swallowing difficult, if not impossible.
3. An otitis media (middle ear infection) with heat in the ears, throbbing pain, and bulging (swollen) tympanic membrane (ear drum).
4. A nursing mother with a breast infection. The area is red, swollen, hot and painful, and filled with pus.
5. Meningitis with a high fever of 105°F, a bursting headache which throbs and an inability to fully bend the neck as the meninges are inflamed.

Belladonna is needed in all the above. It is searching for itself in each condition. The cardinal points of inflammation are the guiding symptoms of *Belladonna.* In each of the above conditions, **the name of the disease is irrelevant** for the homeopath, whereas for the allopath it is essential.

The allopath would treat each of the above conditions differently. No. 1 would receive analgesics, No. 2 an antibiotic, and No. 3 an antibiotic and an analgesic. No. 4 would use warm compresses to the area and probably antibiotics as well. No. 5 would be hospitalized with antibiotics if bacterial, analgesics and intravenous fluids.

The homeopath, on the other hand, would only see *Belladonna* and *Belladonna* would cure in each of the above, including meningitis though the prudent homeopath would give *Belladonna* **and** send the patient to the hospital.

In a nutshell, the way a homeopath uses homeopathic *Belladonna* is the way we use all our medicines. We look to find the pathogenetic (proving) symptoms of the medicine in the patient.

Caution! Under no circumstances attempt to treat possible meningitis at home. Always be prudent. Only the most highly skilled homeopath can successfully treat meningitis and even he would send the patient on to the hospital. If he has prescribed correctly, the patient will be discharged quickly. If not, the patient can receive conventional treatment. Also, know that *Belladonna* is but one of many medicines indicated in the treatment of meningitis.

In the next chapter, we'll take a look at unusual symptoms, i.e., those symptoms that are unexpected and inexplicable and most interest the homeopath. These unusual symptoms can often lead to the correct medicine.

seven

Searching For The Strange, The Rare, The Peculiar

The homeopathic physician goes into extreme detail when talking to and observing his patients. Hahnemann urged us to do so. In paragraph 95 of the *Organon* he writes:

> In chronic diseases the investigation of the signs of disease…must be pursued as carefully and circumstantially as possible, and the most minute peculiarities must be attended to, partly because in these diseases they are the most characteristic and least resemble those of acute diseases, and if a cure is to be effected they cannot be too accurately noted.

He goes on to note that patients become so accustomed to their condition that they do not pay attention to small details. It is just these minutiae, says Hahnemann,

> …which are often very pregnant with meaning (characteristic) [and] often very useful in determining the choice of the remedy.

Here Hahnemann, in his words, is talking about **strange, rare and peculiar** symptoms. Let's look at a few of the many rare and peculiar symptoms:

- A patient with acute hepatitis might report he cannot lie on his left side as the liver pain intensifies, but will lie on his right side as the liver pain diminishes. The medicine, *Bryonia,* has to be considered.

- A patient says his headache is pressing like a band around his forehead. *Sulphur* is a strong candidate.
- A woman reports that her sexual desire is much higher during her menses. The medicine, *Pulsatilla,* comes to mind.
- A patient with a stroke says the paralyzed limb feels as though ants were crawling on it. We would have to consider *Phosphorus.*
- A person with severe headaches notes they always come on before a thunderstorm. At least five homeopathic medicines must be taken into consideration.
- Another says she becomes irritable in extreme heat. Many medicines have this feature with *Natrum carbonicum,* the leader.
- A nursing mother reports pain in the breasts only while nursing. *Croton tiglium, Pulsatilla,* and *Silica* have to be considered.

There are literally thousands of peculiar symptoms like these and they can be amazingly helpful in selecting the **simillimum** (most similar medicine).

BACK PAIN RELIEVED WITH HIS WIFE STANDING ON HIS BUTTOCKS

In my practice my ears are constantly attuned for any unusual details that will lead me to the correct medicine. One case involved Cosmo (not his real name), a burly 49-year-old Greek immigrant. He was changing a tire one day in 2002. As he lifted the tire he felt a sudden severe pain in the left side of his lower back. He found that with rest and some non-steroidal anti-inflammatory drugs (NSAIDs) the situation improved within two weeks. However, it was back again when he came to see me in November, 2007. The pain went from the left lumbosacral area to the left hip. He also said that lying on his back was unbearable. "My hamstrings feel like they are moving," he said. To get relief he sometimes punched the area with his fist. "But what gives me the greatest relief," he said, "is for me to lie on my stomach and my wife to stand on either the buttocks or the hamstrings."

Now *that* caught my attention. I had heard of pressure relieving pain but having the wife stand on the buttocks? I wanted to know how much she weighed. "She's around two hundred and thirty pounds," he said. Now that's some pressure!

He said the hamstrings were both restless and tight. "When she steps on them, the relief is tremendous. The pleasure of that release is so great I fall asleep right away." (I know his wife. Since then, she dieted and lost eighty pounds.)

Cosmo disliked sleeping in a bed on a mattress and two years earlier switched to sleeping on the bare floor. "The hard floor pressing up against the sides of my thighs feels good," he said. "Sometimes I'll sit on the edge of a table and the pressure of the table against the back of my thighs feels good."

Can you begin to make sense of Cosmo's problem? That's right. He had muscle pain in the buttocks and hamstrings which was **better from hard pressure**. Very hard pressure. This was not the usual muscular pain that yields to a good massage. No. This pain only yielded to EXTREME pressure. How else to explain sleeping on the floor or a two hundred and thirty pound woman standing on his buttocks?

The homeopath pays attention, first and foremost, to symptoms that are out of the ordinary, and Cosmo's pain and release from pain, were certainly out of the ordinary.

The medicine I was thinking of, *Colocynthis* or Bitter Cucumber, is often associated with anger so I asked him about anger.

"Yes," he said, "I get angry every day. I used to kick garbage cans and throw chairs." He was the owner of a gas station that also sold other items. It was located in a rough and tumble neighborhood. He had a relatively high turnover rate of employees, some of whom stole from him and did not take care of the store.

"What pisses me off is people that lie and people who don't respect other people or other people's property," he said. "When I see paper all over the restroom I feel rage."

He added, "I hate stupidity. I hate lack of respect. When I hold my anger in everything gets worse. I feel my eye wanting to pop out of my head."

Cosmo's case revolved around two factors. The first was muscle pain better from very, very hard pressure and the second was frequent and fairly violent anger.

Indeed, he did need *Colocynthis*. What lead to this prescription was not the location of the muscle pain (buttocks and hamstrings) but the strange way he got relief: sleeping on the bare floor, having his wife put all of her weight directly onto his hamstrings, and sitting on the edge of a table. Any modifying influence making a symptom either better or worse we call a **modality**. For Cosmo, the great modality was "better from hard pressure." He was also an angry person and in the proving of *Colocynthis,* many provers reported feeling strong anger. In fact, in the originally proving conducted by Hahnemann, the following symptom is recorded: "Extreme peevishness; everything is amiss; he is extremely impatient; everything vexes him…" Cosmo got a dose of *Colocynthis.*

When seen again four weeks later, the left lumbosacral pain and the left hip pain had gone away. The hamstrings were no longer moving and twitching. Nor were they painful. His wife had had to stand on the hamstrings but once. His anger had also declined.

"Yeah, now that you mention it," he said, "I fired an employee the other day. She had been stealing and I was totally calm the whole time. That was unusual."

Cosmo was still sleeping on the bare floor. "But now, in the middle of the night, I'll wake and go to bed. Before, I slept all night on the floor."

He was off to a good start. His strange muscle pains were gone. He had received two doses of *Colocynthis* both within a 24-hour period. Contrast this to the treatment he would have received from conventional medicine: a muscle relaxant, possibly an anxiolytic (anti-anxiety medicine) plus pain medicine, all of which he would have had to taken daily for a long time, possibly forever.

It has been over seven years since Cosmos was treated with *Colocynthis* for that pain. He has needed no further treatments for it.

Homeopathy. It's almost like magic. Remember the devil's in the details.

eight

Isopathy – Cousin To Homeopathy

So far, we have been learning how the homeopathic medicine most **similar** to the illness cures that illness. This is the **Law of Similars**. There is a variation on homeopathy and that is **isopathy**. **Iso**- is a Greek prefix meaning, **identical**. When a person has become sick from exposure to a noxious or poisonous substance, it is possible to remove that substance with the same noxious substance in its **potentized** form (Chapter 2). Therefore, a noxious substance that has been **diluted** and **succussed** can remove that same substance in its toxic form. It's the same idea as "Hair of the dog," i.e., when you drink a little alcohol the morning after to lessen the effects of a hangover.

HOMEOPATHY AND DETOXIFICATION

The idea of detoxification is attractive because human beings are exposed to so many toxic substances. Our society is chemically polluted. Non-organic foods are grown with pesticides and herbicides and find their way into our bodies. And that's just the beginning. There are additional tens of thousands of chemicals, many of which are capable of damaging our health.

It is widely known that modern man lives in a sea of toxic chemicals. These are absorbed via the skin, the lungs, and the gut, finding their way into the blood stream where they are transported to various organs and cells. As they accumulate, they can cause damage. It is thought the liver and fat cells end up with most of these toxic chemicals though no organ is immune from their destructive influence. When the body can no longer effectively eliminate these toxins, it falls sick.

The idea, say those who advocate detoxifying the body, is to rid the cells and organs of these toxic wastes via a multitude of cleanses. Colonic therapy (super enemas in which large of amounts of water are injected into the colon and then expelled) has its own set of proponents and practitioners. Then there are others who advocate gallbladder cleanses, liver cleanses, heavy metal cleanses, even ways to rid the body of radioactivity. Most internists and family practitioners pay scant attention to the possibility that their patients could be suffering from toxic buildup. There are exceptions: doctors involved in industrial or occupational medicine are acutely aware of the dangers of toxic chemicals.

The question for us is: can homeopathic medicines remove toxic wastes? There is evidence they can. What follows is a report of arsenic poisoning in an orchard worker. It took place in England nearly eighty years ago. I located the article in its republished form in the June, 1978 issue of *The Layman Speaks*, a homeopathic publication for lay homeopaths that is no longer in existence.

Specific High Potency Homœopathic Remedies
For Heavy Metal Poisoning
by Harold J. Wilson, M.D.

> In 1932 it was my privilege to study under Sir John Weir of London, England. Sir John Weir was the Royal Physician, and one of the leading homoeopaths of that time. During one of his lectures, he told us that a single dose of 1M to 10M of the specific substance that was causing the symptoms would allow the body to expel the offending material quickly and easily.
>
> My first experience with this principle was in 1936, just after my return from 4 years of missionary work in Africa. A 42-year-old orchardist staggered into my office and collapsed on the couch in the waiting room. He was cyanotic; he was perspiring profusely; and his pulse was too rapid to count.
>
> "Doc," he said, "I'm dying."
>
> I was inclined to agree with him! As an apple grower, he had many small exposures to arsenic over the past 20 years. While working

inside a spray tank, he finally received sufficient additional exposure to throw him into an acute toxic condition. Knowing he would never live long enough to make it to the hospital, I stood next to him feeling quite helpless. Suddenly I recalled the lessons of Sir John Weir. From some remedies brought back from London, I found a 10M potency of arsenic (*Arsenicum album*) and poured half a teaspoon of these granules on his tongue. Within an hour, his pulse began to slow down but he still perspired freely. An hour later I was startled to hear him call me. Arriving quickly at his side, he pointed to a white powder that was appearing where the perspiration was drying on the folds of his blue shirt. As he brushed it off, he smelled it and then tasted it.

"This is white arsenic, Doc," he said. "There is enough here to kill three men!"

It seems the one dose of homoeopathic arsenic changed the body's polarity enough so that the toxic arsenic which had been attracted to the cells was now being expelled. Within three hours the patient was able to drive home and was soon completely recovered. He lived the next 41 years of his life free of any further episodes of arsenic toxicity.

I recall this experience to illustrate a simple and practical law of healing. If you know what poison or toxic substance is causing the illness and give a high potency preparation of that substance, you will enable the body to cure itself. This applies to lead, copper, mercury, aluminum, poison ivy, ragweed, and many other substances to which the human body may react in a toxic manner.

TOO GOOD TO BE TRUE?

The above incident reads more like a "tale" than a case report. The *Arsenicum album* acted so fast and so profoundly that it apparently snatched the orchardist from the jaws of certain death and then allowed him to live another forty-one years with nary a recurrence. Clearly, this was an outstanding, if not miraculous, cure. Can homeopathy really be that simple and effective?

In the last paragraph Doctor Wilson suggested that all manner of toxins (lead, copper, mercury, aluminum, poison ivy, ragweed, etc.) can be removed by using the toxic substance in a homeopathic preparation, a most appealing proposition. This method of treatment, as mentioned above, is known as **isopathy** whereby one treats with the identical substance, not the most similar as in homeopathy. In isopathy the offending substance, be it a food, a chemical, a venom, or any poison, is potentized, i.e., made into a homeopathic medicine and given to the patient. This isopathic preparation will then remove the offending poison or allergen and the patient will recover. Isopathy is appealing mainly because it seems direct and easy.

For example, if the patient gets diarrhea every time he drinks milk, you simply potentize milk and give it to him and expect the milk allergy to disappear. It's the same for corn or wheat or peanuts, heavy metals, all pollens, molds, noxious plants such as poison ivy or venoms of snakes, spiders, bees or wasps. Simply dilute and success the harmful substance until it is **potentized** and administer.

Many lay homeopathic practitioners cite cures of poison ivy by using homeopathic *Rhus toxicodendron* (Latin for poison ivy). Yes, it can cure poison ivy, but often it does not. The repertory, *Synthesis,* cites thirty homeopathic medicines known to successfully cure poison ivy, one of which is *Rhus toxicodendron.*

The same caveat applies to all poisonings and intoxications and all allergies. Isopathic preparations can help, but often they do not. The isopathic approach is seductive because it is so simple and it does not require the endless attention to detail or the close inferential reasoning that homeopathy does.

So although those of us who are dyed-in-the-wool homeopaths may occasionally foray into isopathy, we soon revert to homeopathy. As mentioned above, **homeo-** a prefix from the Greek, **homoios**, means similar. It does not mean identical, not **iso-**, a Greek prefix meaning **equal**, as in isopathy.

In homeopathy we are trying to find the most similar medicine, the one in its pathogenesis (proving) that best matches all the symptoms of the patient. Remember: in homeopathy we are taking into account not only the chief complaint, but all the secondary and tertiary ones too. It's a complex undertaking.

But it is important not to minimize the case of the arsenic-intoxicated orchardist who, after receiving *Arsenicum album* 10M, expelled visible arsenic powder on his blue shirt, and did so within three hours of receiving the homeopathic arsenic! The question is: was this result a fluke or is there other evidence that isopathy works?

THE ALUMINUM CONNECTION

A family member suffering from severe allergies to numerous pollens and dust, as well as various foods, had been chronically ill with sinusitis occurring four to five times a year requiring antibiotics and prednisone. In addition, she was asthmatic needing two different inhalers containing steroids, one inhaled into the lungs twice a day, the other into the nostrils once a day. She had very little sense of taste or smell.

At 75-years of age, she had been treated with homeopathy repeatedly by me as well as famous homeopaths from around the world. No homeopathic medicine had acted. She was discouraged; I was discouraged. The great passion of my life, homeopathy, had apparently failed.

Then, in October, 2012, during a conference in which Miranda Castro, a homeopath from Florida, was presenting a case of homeopathic aluminum, known as *Alumina*, she mentioned that black tea contained substantial amounts of aluminum. I went online to discover that if lemon or lime was added to black tea the absorption of aluminum went up six fold. My patient had come to me nearly thirty years ago. At that time, I told her to stop drinking coffee as I believed, along with most homeopaths, that coffee antidoted homeopathic medicine. (I no longer believe that.) She stopped coffee and immediately started drinking black tea which she steeped for twenty or more minutes every time *and* she added lemon. She had two or three cups a day. So, for twenty-eight years, she had been unwittingly absorbing aluminum via the gut. In addition, for over fifty years, she had used deodorants containing aluminum. Immediately, she stopped both the deodorant and tea and was given *Alumina* which is the homeopathic preparation of aluminum oxide. She took a daily dose of a low potency.

She had been irrigating her nasal passages twice daily with salt and baking soda for nearly two years. It had helped slightly, but she continued to have frequent sinusitis requiring antibiotics and steroids and the asthma continued unabated. As soon as *Alumina* was introduced, her nasal irrigations began to yield all sorts of debris. I say, "debris," because she reported not only discharging masses of slimy, multi-colored mucus, but old blood and tissue as well. These discharges continued for months but from the very start of using *Alumina* she reported feeling much better. Her energy rose, her coughing stopped, and within a month she was off all three steroid inhalers. She has remained asthma free, nor has she had further sinusitis requiring antibiotics or steroids. Her sense of taste and smell remain impaired as of this writing, but the overall improvement has been striking.

Evidently, she was suffering from aluminum toxicity with the aluminum accumulating in the mucous membranes of the sinuses and airways effectively preventing homeopathic medicines, prescribed the usual way, from acting. *Alumina*, in this case, was used *isopathically*.

Interestingly, Hahnemann, in the *Organon*, alluded to something similar. In the third paragraph, he wrote about the qualities that a, "true practitioner of the healing art," needed. I quote from the end of that paragraph:

> ...if he [the physician] knows the *obstacles to recovery* [italics mine] in each case and is aware how to remove them, so that the restoration [of health] may be permanent, *then he understands how to treat judiciously and rationally*...

Aluminum, a recognized neurotoxin, was clearly an **obstacle to cure**.

Since 2012, I have used *Alumina* isopathically in a number of patients in whom I have suspected aluminum toxicity often with surprisingly good results.

We live in the **Age of aluminum**. It is everywhere. As the third most common element after oxygen and silicon, it comprises eight percent of the earth's crust by weight. Despite its ubiquity, it had always remained locked up in combination with other elements and essentially unavailable to human beings. Aluminum is the most abundant metal on earth. It is never found free in nature but is bound to other elements to form compounds. Alum (potassium aluminum sulfate) and aluminum oxide are two of the most common compounds.

Though all animal and eventually human life evolved in a sea of aluminum, the metal had virtually no effect on living things. This all changed in the late nineteenth century when aluminum began to be mined and made into a variety of products. As the twentieth century unrolled, aluminum found its way into more and more materials and products. Though the vast majority of aluminum products are external to human beings and, hence, have no effect on our health, a significant (and growing) amount has found its way into products that are either ingested, applied directly onto the skin (sun block, deodorants and antiperspirants), or injected intramuscularly (approximately half of all childhood vaccines contain aluminum) and even intravenously (in neonatal intensive care units, tiny premature babies receive a nutritional compound that contains aluminum).

That aluminum is everywhere is a fact of tremendous import because, **for the first time in human evolution**, aluminum has found its way into many of our organs including our brain. **Aluminum is a neurotoxin**, that is, it literally poisons nerve cells. There is no dispute about its neurotoxicity yet it is sanctioned by the governments of the world and by the medical professions. In the United States, the Food and Drug Administration has designated aluminum as **GRAS** (Generally Regarded As Safe) despite the publication of thousands of scientific articles attesting to its neurotoxicity.

Aluminum is definitely implicated in Alzheimer's Disease though not all researchers believe, as I do, that it is causative. Some believe the aluminum enters the brain because the person already has Alzheimer's. There are a number of investigators who believe aluminum's wide use as an adjuvant in childhood vaccines may be partly or wholly responsible for the rise of autism and the autistic spectrum of diseases (Asberger's, ADHD, ADD).

In my clinical practice, I can only report that in a number of patients, homoeopathic *Alumina* restores memory deficits, improves coordination and boosts energy. Much more work needs to be done in this area by concerned physicians. Aluminum, despite the FDA's labeling it as generally safe, is anything but. It is, purely and simply, a neurotoxin and a dangerous one.

HOMEOPATHIC ARSENIC USED TO TREAT ARSENIC POISONING

A study out of West Bengal, India, showed encouraging results in removing arsenic from two groups of villagers who had been drinking arsenic-contaminated water from tube wells. Chronic exposure to arsenic adversely affects the functioning of the kidneys, liver, lungs, and skin and often the appetite is diminished. Most of the villagers suffered from muscle aches and pains, very low energy and depression.

Subjects in both groups received *Arsenicum album* 30c twice daily for ten consecutive days and urine samples were collected for eleven days. In the second group only, blood samples were also collected and analyzed for arsenic. The investigators found that the amount of arsenic excreted via the urine was much higher than normal in both groups and that it peaked on the seventh day. In the second group blood arsenic showed a significant drop by day 30 and returned to normal by day 60. Many of the villagers, but not all, experienced improvement in their energy, mood, muscle aches and appetite.

The above study was published online October 19, 2005. It can be read in full at ecam.oxfordjournals.org/cgi/reprint/neh124v1pdf

Isopathy could prove useful in hospitals in cases of overdoses. It is common for hospitals to admit moribund patients who have ingested different poisons. Treating those patients isopathically could improve their chances of survival.

PART II

Testimony of the clinic

Part I discussed the principles and philosophy of homeopathic medicine. To fully understand homeopathy requires a paradigm shift. All homeopaths make this paradigm shift because homeopaths treat the person with the disease, not the disease in the person.

In Part II, the focus is on the clinic and illustrates how the principles, thus far elucidated, are put to use in the treatment of sick folks. What follows in Part II are examples of medical disorders that have shown remarkable improvement using homeopathic medicines. They have been selected not only because the results have been outstanding but also because they illustrate homeopathic principles.

Many books on homeopathy attempt to group clinical conditions (of the heart, lung, gastrointestinal, nervous system, or the skin, etc.) and show which homeopathic medicines are useful in each condition. This is a mistaken approach as we are treating the person *and* his disease rather than just the disease. We shall focus, as Dr. Prafull Vijayakar, a well-known Indian homeopath says, on "Man in disease rather than disease in man."

Instead, cases will be presented that demonstrate one medicine acting in quite different pathological conditions as well as how one condition can be treated with different homeopathic medicines.

The reason is that we are looking for the **simillimum** which is that medicine which most perfectly corresponds (is most similar) to the person who is ill as well as the symptoms he or she is presenting.

The cases presented cover a small sample of illnesses and pathological conditions that homeopathic medicine is capable of addressing.

nine

How Important Is A Diagnosis?

A Case Of Belladonna

In Chapter 3, we looked at how drugs are designed and act and how homeopathic medicines act. The differences are huge. In Chapter 6, we showed how keynote symptoms of *Belladonna* can lead to its use in different clinical situations, each with its own diagnosis. *Belladonna* can also be used in more unusual and complex situations as in the following case.

A thirty-one-year-old woman came in because she could not open her mouth. I did not know that when we sat down in the consulting room. My head was down as I was writing her address and telephone number and I caught myself thinking, "It sounds like she's talking through her teeth," Looking up, I saw she was doing exactly that. Her lips were moving but not her jaw. Her mouth was closed—except for the slight movement of the lips. I was startled at first, then curious.

She said that toward the end of October, 2007, she awoke one day with a tingling sensation in the right side of her face. A few days later, her tongue felt heavy and she began to slur her words. On November 1st, she woke up and was unable to open her mouth. Just like that, her jaw had seized up. "My lips felt paralyzed," she said. "They also felt heavy. So did the right cheek."

She went to the emergency room of a nearby hospital and was admitted for a neurological work up. Computerized tomography (CT) revealed no abnormalities. Her neurologists had NO DIAGNOSIS, and they discharged her.

As her condition did not improve, a couple of weeks later she went to another hospital and was admitted. Magnetic resonance imaging (MRI) of the brain was normal. Again, a second group of neurologists had NO DIAGNOSIS. Again she was discharged.

Two teams of neurologists at two Houston hospitals had said they had never seen anything like whatever it was she had. When I saw her on December 3rd , 2007, she was still unable to move her jaws other than fractionally, though in the past week, some movement and feeling had returned to the lips.

I asked about any past illnesses and she told me she had a seizure disorder that started when she was three years old. She took the antiepileptic drug, *Keppra,* but there was nothing to connect her present inability to open her mouth with epilepsy. She was also under quite a bit of stress but more about that later.

"In 2000, I went in to have my wisdom teeth removed," she said. "The dentist had trouble removing them and several broke off and were left in the sockets." She told her doctors about the wisdom teeth and they thought the fragments of teeth deep in her sockets could be playing a role in her inability to open her mouth. They sent her to an oral surgeon who took a panoramic x-ray of all the teeth and said, in his opinion, that the problem was not due to the teeth. Again, there was NO DIAGNOSIS.

Finally, she was sent to an Ear, Nose and Throat (ENT) specialist who passed a tiny camera up her nose into the back part of the pharynx and decided that the jaw was, "in a state of spasm," but could not say why.

She was discharged, WITHOUT A DIAGNOSIS and without treatment.

She had five children. In 2000, she suffered a miscarriage thought by her doctors possibly to be due to the drug, *Dilantin* that she was taking at the time for her epilepsy. Her fourth child was born with an atrial septal defect, a heart abnormality, and was scheduled for surgery. Another child had a kidney problem.

Often in medicine, stress can lead to emotional and physical problems so I inquired if she had any worries. She said the son with atrial septal defect was also a hemophiliac. For the past year, she had been worrying about him. She got up frequently during the night to check on him. For the past three weeks she had been experiencing sharp pain in the left side of the face two to three inches below the ear that was extending upward. With the pain she had nausea. This morning, before coming to see me, she had sharp, stabbing pains in the right side of the face below the right ear in the jawbone that extended upward. It occurred between four and five o'clock in the morning.

I asked her to describe herself. "I am responsible and active," she said. "I am the team mom. I help on field trips."

She also had two jobs, one at her church for thirty-five hours a week, and the second at a bank, as a teller. She appeared to be very self-contained and self-controlled and said she expected to overcome her current problem. Her husband had been depressed from July to October of that year. "It put a little more strain on me," she said.

I was struck by this woman's aplomb. She appeared able to bear all sorts of responsibilities with hardly a bother. She held two jobs, was an active mom, took a dance class, was active in her children's school and did all this without complaining and without evidence of anxiety or depression. In fact, she seemed quite all right.

At the very end of the interview she said it felt as if her jaw joint was very tight. "I feel the jaw needs to be popped open," she said.

To be very honest, I had quizzed this woman trying to learn if her inability to move her jaws was possibly a hysterical phenomenon. I was satisfied it was not. She could not have been more calm, more centered, or more objective. So I used the physical symptoms and looked them up in my repertory:

- **Cramping & spasm of jaw joints** (she felt it, the ENT confirmed it).
- **Industrious** (she worked two jobs and ran a large family).
- **Benevolent** (she did for others).

Running through those symptoms was *Belladonna* although she did not have any of the cardinal signs of inflammation (redness, heat, swelling, pain and loss of function) that point directly to *Belladonna* as explained in Chapter 6. Yet the three symptoms above pointed unmistakably to *Belladonna.* What I did not mention in Chapter 6 was that in Hahnemann's original proving of *Belladonna,* 1,440 symptoms were recorded and in the repertory I use there are over 11,000 symptoms attributed to *Belladonna*. So *Belladonna* is a hugely multi-faceted medicine and can be used in many different clinical situations.

She was given a single dose of *Belladonna* 200c.

A week or so later, she called to say the spasm of the jaws resolved quickly as did all other symptoms. She was overjoyed and, of course, so was I.

Homeopathic treatment can be successful even without a diagnosis

I report this woman's case for another reason. Though she had no diagnosis and could not be treated by her other doctors, she was easily treated by homeopathy. Note: I, also, had no firm diagnosis. For medical doctors, a diagnosis is considered the indispensable first step. Diagnose accurately, then treat, is a given.

Homeopaths, on the other hand, know that an accurate diagnosis is not always possible. But we can function very well without one because we rely upon the symptoms which, for us, are signposts to the medicine. The symptoms are a reflexion of the disordered Vital Force, according to Hahnemann. LIKE CURES LIKE has very little to do with the diagnosis and EVERYTHING to do with the symptoms. The homeopathic medicine that is most LIKE the symptoms presented by the patient will cure as it did in this case.

COST

This woman saw teams of specialists, each highly paid, and underwent many sophisticated and costly tests. Many thousands of dollars later, she was where she began–with the original problem unresolved. When I contacted her several years later she mentioned how she was still paying down her co-pay. She saw me only one time and paid me a single fee of $260.00. That fee included the homeopathic medicine.

ten

Colic – A Bane Of Babies – And Their Parents!

Baby Anna had been screaming since birth. "She screams uncontrollably from 7 till 11 p.m. or even midnight," said her mother. Anna was her firstborn and I saw her when she was fifteen days old.

When the cry is loud and continuous and lasts one to four hours, often in the evening after feeding, it is called "colic" or "infantile colic" and it is the bane of many young mothers.

Dr. Morris A. Wessel, a clinical professor of pediatrics at Yale Medical School in New Haven, in a 1954 article in *Pediatrics,* referred to this condition as "paroxysmal fussing" or "infantile colic." It occurs in an otherwise healthy and well-fed baby who cries or screams for a good three hours a day, often in the evening. It goes on most days of the week and can last for months.

Colic is thought to be the result of the baby's immature digestive tract which fails to digest mother's milk (or formula) resulting in painful abdominal bloating. The brand new digestive system is literally learning how to process food. Peristalsis, the involuntary constriction and relaxation of the muscles of the stomach and gut which knead the food, sending it down the digestive tract, is thought to be functioning imperfectly resulting in the bolus of food staying too long in the stomach or small intestine. Moreover, the number of beneficial bacteria (*probiotics*) that aid in the breakdown of food are, presumably, inadequate. Sometimes the mother's diet contains foods that she digests and tolerates well but when parts of those foods find their way into her milk, the infant cannot tolerate them setting up a kind of allergic reaction in the child.

Often, the colic is simply unexplainable and mother and child suffer through it until the child's digestive system matures sufficiently and it finally winds down. Colic affects an estimated twenty-five percent of newborns. It can last for four to six months and is stressful for both the baby and the parents who often lose sleep and patience. Some mothers with colicky babies go into high anxiety.

Anna also had a high bilirubin, a breakdown product of hemoglobin, the oxygen-carrying pigment of red blood cells. It is common for bilirubin to be elevated in newborns turning the skin yellow. It is called "physiological jaundice" and can affect up to fifty percent of newborns. Anna's was high enough to concern her pediatrician and she had been admitted to the hospital several times for light therapy to bring it down. Despite the light therapy it jumped back up again. The high bilirubin eventually returns to normal levels in the great majority of babies.

ENTER HOMEOPATHY

As always, I began to search for a homeopathic medicine that corresponded closely to Anna's symptoms and to Anna, the person. I learned that her mother had been drinking a health drink called Noni juice. She had already stopped drinking it, but the colic continued.

Symptoms that I deemed important were:

- Anna's colic was worse lying on her back, and slightly better lying on her right side.
- Her head was quite hot and her feet cold.
- "She is expressive," said her mother. "She already has many facial expressions. She was born at noon and kept her eyes open for the next fifteen hours."

The fact she stayed awake fifteen hours the day of her birth intrigued me. To me, it signified she was a **curious** child, already interested in learning about her new environment and excited to be here.

Based on her friendliness and the fact she was worse lying on her back and better on her right side, I gave *Phosphorus.* Two days later she was no better. Reconsidering, I gave more importance to her curious nature and the fact her head was warm and her feet cold. These symptoms indicated *Sulphur.* She received a single dose and two days later the colic was no more, much to the delight of her parents. Rather than four or more months of suffering, homeopathy cured her colic before she was three weeks old. Oh yes, the bilirubin also dropped to normal which would have happened anyway though the *Sulphur* may very well have speeded up the process.

In order to understand how a homeopath thinks, let us look again at Baby Anna's case. She had infantile colic with all the expected symptoms, what we homeopaths call common symptoms. All babies with colic behave in a similar fashion—prolonged, loud crying for hours a day–that often comes on after feeding. COMMON SYMPTOMS NEVER HELP THE HOMEOPATH FIND THE CORRECT MEDICINE.

Why is that? In the provings (Chapter 3) we find that virtually all homeopathic medicines produce many common symptoms. Most medicines will cause headache, stomach upset, constipation, diarrhea, joint pains, sleeplessness, cheerfulness, sadness, anger, grief, feeling too hot or too cold, etc. If most medicines cause similar, common symptoms we have no means of distinguishing one from the other. Fortunately, in each proving, a number of distinctive symptoms have also been produced, i.e., UNUSUAL SYMPTOMS THAT HAVE COME TO CHARACTERIZE THE MEDICINE AND ENABLE US TO PRESCRIBE. So, in every case of illness, we look for what is uncommon or particular to this particular patient with his or her particular problem.

The fact Anna's colic was worse lying on her back was striking. Not all babies with colic are worse lying on the back. So, for a homeopath, that symptom becomes important. That her head was hot and her feet cold does not occur in all cases of colic, so that also helps to individualize Anna's colic.

And, perhaps most important was the fact that she stayed awake FIFTEEN hours the first day of her life suggesting she was intensely interested in her new world–a very curious child.

These three symptoms called for *Sulphur* which cured her. People who need *Sulphur* tend to be intensely curious. Often they end up making important discoveries in science and technology.

Homeopaths look to those symptoms that are characteristic of the person and distinctive of the illness *and* which correspond to those unusual symptoms produced in the provings.

eleven

Treating A Potentially Dangerous Eye Infection

Herpes simplex, a common virus infecting humans, is known as the cause of cold sores, sometimes called fever blisters, that occur on the lips or around the mouth. Sometimes, the herpes simplex virus attacks the eye targeting the cornea. The infection can be superficial involving the top layer of the cornea. It usually heals without scarring. Sometimes, the virus attacks deeper levels and can lead to scars of the cornea, impaired, or even, loss of vision.

A thirteen-year-old boy developed pain in the left eye twelve days before I saw him. There was redness, swelling and tearing of the eye. "It felt like something was in it, like a speck of dirt" he said. Then his vision blurred. He was taken first to an optometrist who referred him to an ophthalmologist. Neither offered a diagnosis. Finally, a second ophthalmologist diagnosed herpes simplex virus and prescribed oral antibiotics plus ophthalmic antibiotic drops. The parents did not start the antibiotics, preferring that he be treated homeopathically. I saw him in October, 2002.

The left upper lid was swollen and the conjunctiva "injected," meaning there was redness of the sclera of the eye—a sign of inflammation. The eye was sensitive to light. A lymph node in front of the left temporomandibular joint (TMJ) was swollen and tender to touch. The two eyelids were stuck together in the morning.

All these symptoms are common to inflammation of the cornea and common symptoms are not useful to the homeopath who is always listening and looking for something out of the ordinary.

Suddenly, he came out with it. “A bit earlier it felt as if an object was shoved up under my upper eyelid,” he said. Also, all eye symptoms were worse outside in the open air.

I searched the Repertory and found, “Pain, behind lids, as from a foreign body.” There are five homeopathic medicines listed, one of which is *Mercurius.* I knew *Mercurius* could be effective in inflammation of the cornea including corneal ulcers. I then consulted *Materia Medica Pura* by Samuel Hahnemann, first published in 1811. In the proving of *Mercurius* are the following symptoms:

- “The light of the fire dazzles the eyes greatly.”
- “The eyes cannot bear the light of the fire and daylight.”
- “Inflammation of both eyes, with burning smarting pain; worse in the open air.”
- “The eyelids are stuck together in the morning.”
- “Sensation under the left upper eyelid, as if a cutting body were behind it.”

These symptoms were a perfect description of the boy’s eye problem. He was given homeopathic *Mercurius* in water. He took a few drops a day. Within one day, the eye was fifty percent improved and within two days, nearly normal. He went on to a full recovery. His parents took him back to the ophthalmologist who, in the words of the parents, was “impressed” by the cure.

This case illustrates that homeopathic medicines, when correctly prescribed, act swiftly in severe inflammation. It also shows how the diagnosis of herpes simplex virus affecting the cornea played no role in my prescribing *Mercurius.* I simply took all the symptoms pertaining to the eye or as Hahnemann phrased it, “**the totality of the symptoms**.” The patient’s eye symptoms **matched** the proving symptoms of *Mercurius.* Instead of relying solely on the repertory, I also consulted *Materia Medica Pura,* a compilation of Hahnemann’s original provings. Homeopaths often consult the repertory and one or several materia medicas before finally selecting the simillimum.

LIKE CURES LIKE. It’s the homeopathic way.

twelve

Mental Symptoms – Why They Can Be Crucial

The initial interview with a careful homeopath often lasts one and a half hours, and sometimes longer. In the interview the homeopath listens attentively and then asks the patient to expand on one point or another. In a purely physical case, such as the one that follows, the mental state was all-important.

CASE OF A COUGH THAT WOULD NOT GO AWAY

Everybody has had a cough. They accompany colds and they pass. But every so often a cough does not go away and morphs into an all-consuming torment. Such was the cough of an old patient of mine who called me in the winter of 2009.

He had already been to his local doctor for this same cough and probable bronchitis and had received a Z-pak (antibiotic) and a Medrol pak (steroids). That treatment ended a week earlier but he was no better.

When we spoke, he was complaining of a tickling in the trachea (windpipe) that produced violent coughing. The mucus he expelled was "stringy" he said. He was coughing so hard it was lasting up to one or two minutes. "It's like a spasm," he said. "I've even gagged."

He was feeling dull and lackadaisical. "Just sitting around," he said.

He then began to speak about a deep sadness that had come over him. "I feel kind of homeless since Ike," he said. Ike was the hurricane that slammed Galveston and Houston in September, 2008. He used to live in Galveston and was now further down the coast in Port Aransas.

"Why do you say you feel homeless?" I wanted to know.

"After Ike, I went up north and stayed with my brother and sister-in-law," he said. "But the truth is I feel I am only welcome if there are projects for me to do."

He had done a major project for them. As soon as it was finished he got the strong impression he was no longer wanted and left.

"I've been depressed," he said, "wondering what the point of living is. Some times I feel that nobody loves me."

He was a man in his sixties, a retired prosecutor. "I felt deeply hurt by my brother and sister-in-law," he said.

He was very chilly—not tolerating the cold at all. "I couldn't get warm in St. Louis," he said. "I wore a stocking cap to bed." His head was the part most sensitive to the cold. He reported drooling at night and sweating on the head and the front part of the neck. He had to force himself to drink.

He spoke again about his brother. "I felt very alienated and alone there," he said.

It turned out that wherever he went (he traveled quite a lot since his retirement), he stayed with friends and always helped them out doing various projects. He liked helping others. He was and had always been a diligent person, hard-working and responsible.

He was taking cough medicine to suppress the cough but it wore off in the early morning hours. At that time he would cough for one to two minutes.

There are over two hundred homeopathic medicines for coughs. A classical homeopath will select only one. In order for it to act curatively it has to match the nature of the cough and the nature of the person.

Here we have a patient with a racking cough that had become chronic. Neither antibiotics nor steroids had stopped it. Daily cough medicine suppressed the cough for a few hours and then it returned. Clearly, this cough was refusing to respond to treatments that targeted only the physical level.

However, he was not suffering simply from a cough. He volunteered information about his "deep sadness." He was feeling unloved, unappreciated, and he was extremely chilly. A homeopath must take all key factors into account and the mental symptoms are often the most important.

Hahnemann writes in *Organon*, paragraph 211:

> ...the state of the disposition of the patient often chiefly determines the selection of the homeopathic remedy, as being a decidedly characteristic symptom which can least of all remain concealed from the accurately observing physician.

My analysis was as follows:

- He felt alone, forsaken, and in grief.
- He was benevolent, always helping others.
- He was diligent, a hard, conscientious worker.
- The cough was peculiar in that the more he coughed the worse it got.
- The medicine selected had to be chilly and thirstless.

The medicine I chose, *Ignatia,* is known for its ability to cure a cough that increases in intensity the more one coughs. Also, it is a well-known grief medicine. People needing *Ignatia* are *chilly* and *thirstless* and can enjoy helping others. Within twenty-four hours of taking *Ignatia* he was markedly better and well within two days. Not only did the cough go away, but he became his upbeat, cheerful self again.

Was *Ignatia* treating the cough? Was it treating the sadness? As both were resolved, we can infer it was treating both. Homeopathy makes no strong distinction between mental symptoms and physical symptoms. Both represent a disordered Vital Force. As the Vital Force normalizes with the correct homeopathic medicine, the physical and mental symptoms diminish and disappear. As I present other cured cases, it will become more evident that the mind and body are a unit and must be treated as a unit for a true cure to occur.

thirteen

Warts

Everyone hates warts. They are unsightly, even disfiguring. They are caused by viruses that invade the outer layer of the skin causing keratin, a hard protein in the epidermis, to grow too fast. These hard, tough cells push up and out, forming a wart. These viruses belong to the human papillomavirus family (HPV) and more than one hundred different ones have been identified.

The cure of warts is a mix of folklore, old wives' tales, and urban legend. Medical science has a number of treatments which include external applications such as salicylic acid and cantharidin. Some dermatologists apply liquid nitrogen to freeze the warts. They can also be burned out, lasered out, or cut out.

A small girl, almost four years of age, had three fairly good-sized warts on her fingers. Her mother had taken her to two pediatric dermatologists and one regular dermatologist. Freezing had failed, as well as injecting a blistering agent. When her mother brought her to me she had been told she would need to have them surgically cut out.

I was not surprised that the dermatologists' treatments had failed. They were treating an internal disease, in this case a virus, with external treatments. Homeopaths are universally opposed to such treatments. The wart is the end result of the virus. The only way to treat a wart is to treat the person with the wart, as well as anything unusual about the wart.

The fact her warts were all on her fingers was striking, as relatively few homeopathic medicines are known to treat warts appearing only on the fingers. Also, she liked salty chips and was a kindly child. She shared with other children and liked to take care of her older brother and her baby sister. "She is very sweet to her baby sister who is three months old," said her mother.

I took the following rubrics:

- Warts on fingers.
- Desire for salt.
- Sympathetic.

The medicine was *Causticum.* She received a single dose and in the next thirty days the warts got smaller and smaller and disappeared. They were cured from within.

How elegant! Rather than assailing the warts with crude chemicals from without, the body cured itself with a gentle nudge from *Causticum* taken by mouth.

Causticum is one of three homeopathic medicines that are famous for removing warts. The others are *Thuja occidentalis* and *Nitric acid.*

All the homeopathic books mention these medicines and many homeopaths give them in a routine sort of way. However, that is NOT homeopathy. There are no specifics in homeopathy. As a result, those three medicines only sometimes remove warts.

Why is this? It is because we treat the disease THROUGH THE INVIDIVIDUAL. It is the individual who is producing the warts. Each individual is unique with unique characteristics and these characteristics have little to do with the wart. In the above case, the little girl's extremely sympathetic nature plus her desire for salt and the location of the warts (fingers) pointed to *Causticum* which cured.

Let's look at another person with warts who did not receive one of the three famous wart medicines.

A fourteen-year-old boy came to me in March, 2005, with warts on his fingers near his nails. Several years earlier, he had warts on the soles of his feet. They had been burned off by a dermatologist.

This is NOT the way to treat warts. They are NOT a local, external disease. Yes, they do appear on the exterior. Yes, they do localize on the skin. But, they can only be there because of the cooperation of the whole organism. Nothing occurs without the permission of the larger whole. The virus cannot take root and grow the wart unless conditions permit.

It's a bit like growing orchids. They need the right soil, the right temperature, and the right mixture of sun and shade. All factors together permit orchids to grow. Without these right conditions the orchids cannot thrive.

So it is with warts. If you burn them off, they will grow back either in that spot or elsewhere. Best to make the internal milieu so strong and healthy that the virus that makes the wart cannot survive.

I discovered this teenager was hot-natured, i.e., he had good body heat and preferred cooler weather. He uncovered in bed at night. He regularly had a bowel movement immediately on rising in the morning.

He also described, "An empty sensation in the stomach." It occurred daily around 11 a.m.

Now, that is striking! When I searched for that symptom in the Repertory, the leading medicine under the heading, "STOMACH, Emptiness, morning, 11 a.m." is *Sulphur*. It happens that people who need *Sulphur* are warm-natured and prefer the cool and tend to have their bowel movement immediately or soon after rising.

Notice! I paid scant attention to the wart. Rather, I paid attention to the **totality of the symptoms**. Here, the totality was:

- Hot-natured. He uncovered at night.
- Bowel movement immediately on rising.
- Empty sensation in the stomach at 11 a.m.

All these qualities or characteristics of the boy are also characteristics of *Sulphur*. After a single dose, the warts slowly receded and ceased growing in the next two to three months. Four and a half years later, I saw him for another problem and learned the warts had never come back.

fourteen

Arnica Montana

Arnica montana is the number one homeopathic medicine for trauma affecting soft tissue, i.e., the bruising and the swelling that accompany it. People who know only one homeopathic medicine know *Arnica*. It is the first medicine in sports injuries and has enabled many an athlete to recover quickly from a fall, a blow or a kick. In recent years a number of plastic surgeons have begun to use *Arnica* post-operatively to control swelling and discoloration following cosmetic surgeries. Every medicine cabinet should contain *Arnica*. Three small pellets constitute a dose and one or two doses a day for two or three days are usually sufficient. *Arnica* can be used after major surgery to control pain and swelling.

Arnica also can be effective in more complex medical problems. The proving symptoms of *Arnica* show that it affects the mind as well as the body. The following example involved a nasty land feud that ended up causing extreme physical pain and mental anguish.

A seventy-year-old woman, a self-confessed workaholic, came in complaining of extreme pains in her left upper arm and, to a lesser extent, in the right upper arm. She said the areas were "hard and painful." Recently, she had been gardening. It involved bending over planting seeds, also pulling weeds. These simple maneuvers, which she had been doing for many years, were no longer possible because of the pain.

"It feels like someone is ripping my arm off," she said. "All the muscles are being ripped."

Also, the left heel felt as if "bruised by a stone." She could not step on it without pain. She could not lie on either side because, she said, "The pain is excruciating." In addition, her boss had been cutting back on her hours and she felt she was being forced out of her job, a job she had been performing faithfully and well for many years.

I had known her for over ten years. She was entirely accustomed to hard physical work and was, if anything, something of a stoic who rarely complained of anything so for her to use "ripping" to describe her pain caught my attention.

I asked if anything else stressful had occurred in her life recently.

"Yes, the worst thing in our whole lives…it's about our land," she said.

She and her husband lived and farmed trees on twenty-three acres in East Texas. Eleven of the acres her husband had inherited. The other twelve had been deeded to him by his great uncle and aunt. Her husband had been living on the land for sixty-nine years. He discussed the deed with a title company. These twelve acres had been part of forty acres. This uncle had a gambling problem and sold twenty-eight acres to settle a gambling debt. That was in 1946.

With the title company's comments attached, he filed the deed in the local county courthouse. Sometime later, a survey team appeared on their property. Her husband, not suspecting anything, allowed them to proceed. It turned out another party was laying claim to his land. The survey was grossly inaccurate. He protested and one day a swarm of off-duty law enforcement officers entered his land and belligerently asked him, "What right do you think you have to this land?" Another threatened to grab him out of his living room and take him to jail.

He stood his ground. He was certain these off-duty lawmen had been hired to intimidate him. Eventually, they left but a few days later a bulldozer appeared on his property and brazenly bulldozed down shrubs and trees on three to four acres right in the center of his twelve acres.

The other party started a lawsuit claiming his land was theirs. He counter-sued. The matter was being adjudicated when I saw her.

I asked my patient how she was reacting to having her land unlawfully surveyed, having corrupt law enforcement officials threaten her and her husband and having her land entered and bulldozed. "It has been absolutely the worst thing to happen to us in our whole lives," she said. She felt she was confronting supremely evil people and feared they might possibly succeed in their efforts to take their land.

She volunteered, "It feels like I've been beaten within an inch of my life." Though she was describing her bodily pains, it was an apt metaphor for the way the other party had been abusing her and her husband.

She was to receive *Arnica montana* though she had suffered no physical trauma. Yet she felt as though she had been "beaten with an inch of my life." People needing *Arnica* often say they feel "bruised" and "sore" and, sometimes, "beaten." The bruised, sore, beaten feeling can result, not only from trauma but also from financial loss and the perceived threat of evil.

In *Materia Medica Pura* by Samuel Hahnemann, in the section describing the effects of *Arnica* it is written: "Fears; anxious dread of coming evil." That means that at least one prover, after taking *Arnica,* reported experiencing a dread of impending evil.

Though the physical symptoms of *Arnica* are well-known, few homeopaths are aware that *Arnica* can be of use when confronted with stark evil. Examples: female children in bed at night afraid of a male figure coming to abuse them; fear of a terrorist bombing; fear of torture, etc., etc.

It is important that the physical sensations of *Arnica,* that is, the bruised, beaten feeling, the ripped apart sensation, be present along with the "anxious dread of coming evil." In addition, my patient and her husband were under financial strain because of the litigation.

She received a single dose of *Arnica* in the 1000 potency (diluted 1000 times).

The next day she called to say she had the worst headache of her life. I told her it would pass. Often patients experience a worsening of symptoms before the improvement starts. Homeopaths refer to such a response as an **aggravation**. Sure enough, the next day she was beginning to improve. Within two to three days, she was back at work though still unable to lift heavy objects.

When I saw her three weeks later, she reported feeling seventy-five to eighty-five percent better.

"I was really bad when I saw you three weeks ago," she said. "That pain was excruciating. It was like, 'Please, God, take my life.'

"You know, within minutes of taking *Arnica* my feeling of hopelessness disappeared. It made me feel like a human being again. I was feeling like a poor little donkey they beat until he falls down in the mud."

Her report of immediate improvement deep in herself is important. A true cure should begin with a sense that the patient has improved in her core. Then the physical symptoms will follow. Hers decreased markedly day by day. "The pain is not nearly as intense as it was," she reported. "Now it is more of a dull pain. Also, I can now lie on either side. Before, I could only lie flat on my back."

I asked about her emotional state. "It is much better. I was really, really depressed when I saw you," she said. "I'm a lot more cheerful now and not so worried about the land."

This case illustrates how a long-standing fearful situation can result in unbearable musculoskeletal pains. By treating this woman's anguish **and** her sensation that she had been beaten as a single phenomenon, *Arnica* was able to successfully resolve both.

Her husband was not so fortunate. Though at the time, he appeared unfazed by the land dispute, he developed an unrelenting cough. Homeopathic treatment was unsuccessful. A chest x-ray revealed a cancer of the lungs. Despite radiotherapy and chemotherapy, he died within two months of the diagnosis.

MORE ON 'DREAD OF COMING EVIL'

It was some years back that I first "discovered" what Hahnemann had found out over two hundred years ago, i.e., that *Arnica* could cure an irrational fear of pending evil. A woman in her forties came in to my clinic on September 19, 2002, complaining of low energy, frequent weeping with depression. Two months earlier, she had had a splenectomy (removal of the spleen). "I'm scared I won't be able to pay my bills," she said. She was not sleeping well. "I'm up all night. I can't stop thinking of all my obligations."

She said she was tossing and turning all night. Most people, when they hear that a person with sleep problems is tossing and turning, accept it as a common consequence of sleeplessness. Not a homeopath. We always want to know why as people toss and turn in bed for different reasons.

"Why do you toss and turn?" I asked.

"I try to find a comfortable position. It may feel right for a few minutes and then it doesn't. I'm uncomfortable and then I have to find a new position." She was speaking in code. She didn't know she was speaking in code, but I did. She was saying that the reason she kept shifting her position was because her body felt uncomfortable, even sore, when it stayed in one position too long. A bit later, she confirmed my hunch when she said, "My bed feels hard. I can't get comfortable." Again, she was speaking in code. Her bed, which she had been sleeping in for years, had not changed. But she had. Her body was sore and, to her, the bed felt "hard."

She also mentioned she had been irritable, quarreling with her mother. Sudden noise caused her to start.

I considered everything she was saying and concluded she needed either *Rhus toxicodendron* or *Arnica* because both medicines have the sensation that the bed feels too hard.

I opened *Materia Medica Pura* and began reading the proving of *Arnica* when I came across, "Fears; anxious dread of coming evil."

"Do you have any fear that something evil could happen?" I asked.

She gasped, "How did you know? Yes, at night I think the terrorists are coming and are going to break in my house. I live near an airstrip and I have this fantasy that they are going to land and take me hostage."

It had been a year and eight days since 9/11 but for her the terrorist threat was imminent. She needed *Arnica* and she needed it now. She received the 200th potency. When I saw her next, the irrational fear had departed and the bed no longer felt "hard." *Arnica* had helped her body and her mind.

fifteen

Homeopathic Arsenicum In A Drug-Induced Psychosis

The orchardist (Chapter 8) had been exposed to arsenic and was dying. *Arsenicum album* saved him. Here follows an entirely different use of *Arsenicum album*, again demonstrating the scope of our medicines.

A seventy-two-year-old man had knee surgery. When he woke after surgery, his personality had totally changed. Whereas before he was a mild-mannered Dr. Jekyll, now he was a raging and paranoid Mr. Hyde. Though the anesthetic had long worn off, his new persona was alarming the entire nursing staff as well as his wife and step-daughter who called me seven days later exclaiming that her step-father's behavior had become bizarre and frightening.

"He is sleeping all day and is awake all night," she said.

"He yells at my mother and accuses her of all sorts of outrageous things."

"Like what?"

"He says, 'You're not taking care of me. You're trying to get rid of me, to kill me.' It's nonsense. She's doing nothing of the kind."

He was swearing at the nurses and sometimes hitting them. The nurses were trying to get him to do physical therapy but he would have none of it.

"Have you visited him?"

"Yes. I've heard him say he's in prison. He'll say, 'Everyone wants to kill me.' Things like that."

"Is he restless?" I wanted to know.

"Yes. Very. He can't be still."

"Anything else?"

"Well, yes. He insists that my mother stay close by his side even though he treats her abominably."

His thirst had decreased considerably.

"Before the operation was he an angry man?"

"Never. He never behaved this way before. Never," she said. "Sometimes now he just talks gibberish."

Such extreme behavior suggested a psychotic break. He had become insanely paranoid with delusions. Presumably, it was the effect of the anesthesia.

His behavior was fully consistent with the homeopathic medicine, *Arsenicum album.* In the repertory are the following rubrics, all containing *Arsenicum album.* I have listed the many rubrics to give an idea of how rich and detailed the Repertory is.

- Thoughts - control of thoughts lost.
- Suspicious, people are plotting against his life.
- Delirium - nonsense, with eyes open.
- Delusions, there are conspiracies against him.
- Delusions, he will be murdered.
- Insanity, desires to escape.
- Insanity, with restlessness.
- Slander - disposition to.
- Speech, unintelligible.
- Speech wild.
- Speech wandering.
- Cursing.
- Foolish behavior.
- Striking.
- Anxious restlessness.
- Fear of being alone.
- Company, desire for.
- Sleeplessness, night.

A few hours later, after a single dose of *Arsenicum album*, he reverted to his old self. There were no relapses and he had an uneventful recovery and was discharged.

"It was fantastic the way it worked," said his step-daughter.

In this situation *Arsenicum album* was prescribed because it was the most similar medicine. There was no evidence of arsenic intoxication as there was in the case of the orchardist.

It is important to understand that this particular case of *Arsenicum album* represents only **one facet** of the medicine, a facet that most homeopaths have never seen. Most patients needing *Arsenicum* do not present this way as illustrated by the orchardist (Chapter Eight) and in the case that follows in the next chapter.

(The above incident occurred in November, 2000. The case was taken by phone.)

sixteen

Post Traumatic Stress Disorder Resolved with Homeopathic Arsenic

Post-traumatic stress disorder (PTSD) is a severe anxiety disorder that can develop after serious injury with the threat of imminent death. Commonly, the person with PTSD describes re-experiencing horrific images of the traumatic event, nightmares of the event or reactions to situations that remind the person of the event.

It is strongly associated with soldiers returning from combat in Iraq and Afghanistan. However, any traumatic incident can trigger it. These include exposure to natural disasters such as floods or fires, an assault, domestic abuse, rape, or a motor vehicle accident. Those people who arrive first at an accident–policemen, firemen, ski patrollers and paramedics, known as **First responders**, are prone to develop PTSD.

What follows is an unusual, even atypical, example of PTSD.

A sixty-two year old retired merchant marine captain was thrown thirty feet in the air when his motorcycle struck a Mercedes, September 15, 2010. When he hit the car he went unconscious.

He had been on a long road trip and was hurrying–hoping to get home a day early and surprise his wife. "I was trying to make time," he admitted. "I felt driven to get home early."

Fortunately for him, he was wearing full motorcycle gear including a Kevlar suit. Kevlar is a synthetic that is five times stronger than steel on an equal weight basis. It likely saved his life. As it was, he fractured seven ribs, and a huge hematoma, a localized swelling filled with blood, formed on his left thigh. Surgery to drain the hematoma was done in the trauma unit and he was discharged with a Jackson-Pratt drain in the site and an appointment to see a surgeon in his home town. Approximately ten days later, the site became infected with Staphylococcus aureus. Intravenous antibiotics did not control the infection and he was operated on. The wound was debrided, that is, surgically cleaned, and a tube placed. A pump was connected to the tube to assist drainage. The wound then began to heal.

The day following the surgery his wife visited him and found him sitting on the bed weeping. He told her he was weeping, “for all the sadness in the world and all the people who are suffering.”

I spoke to him by phone later that day, October 21st. “When night comes, fear comes,” he said. “Fear of death. Killing and maiming. Rocks falling on people. Slow death. All the world is full of rocks falling. There is war. Arrows everywhere–piercing flesh. I think about all the soldiers who died in wars in the past with wounds similar to mine.”

He went on and on, describing scenes of horror. “I’m much better if J (his wife) is in the room,” he said.

He was prescribed homeopathic *Phosphorus*, a medicine known to help people suffering from fear. One key aspect of *Phosphorus* is that people who need it are much better having someone, preferably a family member, close by. That night he slept peacefully. He remained better for seven to ten days and then went into an even worse state. Had *Phosphorus* been the correct medicine, he would not have relapsed so quickly.

On November 11th we spoke again. “At night, I don’t want to go to bed,” he said. “I can’t be in bed.”

“Why is that?” I wanted to know.

“I don’t know. The feeling is not good. There is a sense of danger. When I’m up it’s a level 3 or 4 but when I lie down it’s a level 8 or 9. I can’t stay in bed. It’s even worse if I close my eyes. With my eyes closed I feel I lose control of the situation. I become afraid. So, I get up and walk around. I’ll nap in a chair but mostly I stay up watching TV until three o’clock. Finally, I’ll sleep for three hours.”

He went on, “When I go to the shower and stand under the water I’m afraid I’ll drown. If I close my eyes in the shower the situation is much worse. If I drink from a bottle, I fear I’ll choke. What would happen if the water stays in your throat and chokes you? I have become afraid of the possibility of dying. As long as my eyes are open and I'm awake I'm okay."

The thoughts of violence had returned. "I have thoughts of boulders crushing people. I think of people being tortured in the Roman Empire. People being cut and tortured, skeletons lying in graves."

Recently, someone came from his home town and they talked about the old days but all he could think about were all of his friends now dead. He spoke of his mother and father. "I wasn't nice enough to them. The same for fat people. In the past, when I saw fat people, I wondered what was wrong with them. Now I regret that. Now, when I see a three hundred pound person I feel sorry for him. I think how miserable he is with his weight. And there's nothing he can do. And he knows he'll be this way for the rest of his life. And I feel sorry for him.

"Now I am home alone and I feel down. Even when J is here I see her face and I think one day she will die. She will be a skeleton. When I go to the mall and walk around and see all the people shopping I think, 'In fifty years they'll all be dead. They'll be skeletons.'"

He then spoke of a coldness around his heart. "In bed, with my eyes closed, I feel panic and I feel cold water surrounding my heart. I actually have felt that around my heart has become cold. It is physical. I feel as if my heart is surrounded by coldness. The bad feelings…the bad thoughts…they are usually accompanied by coldness around my heart."

At this point, he became overwhelmed. He could speak no more and handed the phone to his wife. In the background I heard him crying, but it was not crying, it was a howling. It was chilling to hear. Clearly, he was in desperate straits.

He had once told me that many years back, in his seafaring days, he had captained freighters. He held me spellbound recounting how he had almost lost a 60,000 ton ship in a storm, gale force 12 on the Beaufort scale, (winds 75 to 95 mph and waves above 46 feet).

At the time, I asked him if he had been afraid. "Not at all," was his reply. And here he was now, consumed by terror and tortured by horrible thoughts. His anguish affected me deeply. I knew I had to help him and struggled with my own fear of not being able to help. I considered all he had said and looked for clues to the homeopathic medicine most likely to help him.

Homeopaths listen for the unusual, the strange. I decided the strangest thing was the very real sensation of **coldness around his heart**. That together with thoughts of death, a tremendous sense of guilt over his past, his restlessness and his fear to go to sleep and an equal fear to be alone, lead me to *Arsenicum album.* He was mailed the medicine and within hours of taking it his restlessness, his anxiety, his fearful thoughts, all dissipated and ceased.

Later, after he had recovered, we spoke about November 11th.

"I remember you howling," I said.

"I was howling," he said. "There was so much pain inside...I couldn't relieve it with a few tears. I had to shout it out. I couldn't sit in a chair and cry quietly."

Captain G's PTSD was unusual in that he did not, as most do, relive the motorcycle accident. His horrific thoughts, though triggered by the accident, were of a violence stretching back into ancient times. Also, unusual was his tremendous sense of guilt and the awakening in him of intense compassion for the suffering of others. That compassion has remained with him.

We have now seen three *Arsenicum album* case reports, one involving poisoning by arsenic, the other a psychotic break induced by anesthesia, and the third the result of PTSD. One homeopathic medicine was able to treat all three patients despite the fact the cause was different in each patient. This was because all had symptoms of *Arsenicum album,* an important homeopathic medicine with nearly twelve thousand symptoms in RADAR, the repertory I use. Learning the key points of even one major homeopathic medicine is a daunting task. I often tell students that learning a homeopathic medicine is a bit like being married. Even after years of being together, you are still learning something new about your spouse.

seventeen

Multiple Problems Solved with One Homeopathic Medicine

Dyslexia, a learning disability that impairs a person's ability to read, can also be improved with homeopathy as the following case report shows. Ironically, Sam was brought in by his mother, not primarily for dyslexia, but for his failure to grow. She was hoping I could give Sam something that would cause a growth spurt.

He was a boy of slight build, born in July, 1996. He weighed 59 ½ lbs. and stood 4 feet, 8 ¾ inches tall. He was definitely small for his age. I saw him first in early April, 2010. He was wearing a frayed, pink baseball cap with the visor curled down sharply on the sides. On the cap were the words: "Don't Mess With Texas" and "I build stuff."

"I'm a builder," he said proudly and quite matter-of-factly.

"What have you built?" I asked.

"I built a cardboard tank," he said. "It is five feet long and four feet wide and there is a turret." According to his father, whom I saw later, this was no ordinary model tank. It was huge. Seth fashioned struts out of cardboard and used bits and pieces of scraps from all over the house and yard to make this tank. Then he painted it. He would stand inside this elaborate construction and walk around pretending to be a tank in war mode.

He had also built a huge model of a Cessna plane that had a seven foot wing span and a fuselage six feet long. It was also very elaborate and well-constructed.

"I like to build what I see in my mind," he said.

He was quite proud of his skills and also mentioned he had repaired an "Airsoft" gun for his brother. (Airsoft guns are replica firearms that propel plastic pellets using either compressed gas or a spring-driven piston.) He had an innocent and straightforward way about him and altogether I found him quite charming.

In addition to his smallish stature, he had significant scoliosis and wore a corrective back brace which he didn't like very much. His mother said he was dyslexic and, when asked to describe exactly what she observed, she said, "He sees his creations in three dimensions in his head and then he draws what he sees or he will build directly from his imagination. When he reads he switches the order of words on the page. When he reads a word like 'cat' he will see a cat in his head. The problem is with small words, like articles, as he cannot see them."

He was having trouble falling asleep and it took him around two hours. He worried about going to any social gathering where there were people he didn't know. "I'm shy about making friends," he said. He disliked being the center of attention. Often, he simply did not know why he felt anxious. He liked to play in the mud.

He had a pet snake called Hobbs and he was utterly at ease with Hobbs despite the fact Hobbs had bitten him six times, once on his face. He was completely unconcerned that Hobbs might be dangerous.

"I should perhaps mention," his mother said, "that he has an older brother, Bob, who works on tug boats and is away for twenty days at a time. Seth tends to stutter more when Bob comes home."

His mother said he was "meticulous" about the way he kept his bedroom. "He is a routinist," she said. "When he gets anxious or very timid, he cannot be reasoned out of it."

The fifth of seven children, Sam was hot-natured and liked cold drinks. He had a strong love of fruit. He even wanted a fruit salad instead of a cake for his birthday!

I was struck by three things: Sam was a routinist. He had an extraordinarily creative mind and he didn't mind being bitten by Hobbs, the snake. To have a pet snake is one thing; not to be bothered in the least when that snake bites you repeatedly, especially when it bites you in the face, is something else. I felt it was misplaced confidence. He should have been concerned. It lead me to the *Baryta* group of medicines. People who need *Baryta* often have a habit or manner that is inappropriate and they are routinists. Because he was hot-natured and so imaginative I chose one of the iodides.

Sam received a single dose of *Baryta iodatum.*

When I saw him two months later he was sleeping better and falling asleep quickly. “I know he must be because he no longer comes into our bedroom to complain about not falling asleep,” his mother reported.

His weight at 59 ½ lbs. was unchanged. But his height was now 4’ 9 ½–a gain of ¾ inch! In only two months!

I asked him to read aloud and he did so quite fluently. “This is amazing,” his mother said. His father concurred. “This boy was profoundly dyslexic,” he said.

“Also, he is exhibiting a boldness that has surprised me and my husband,” his mother said. “Another thing, he is taking more responsibility. We have a sailboat and he is doing much more to look after it.” When his older brother, Bob, came home, his stuttering was less noticeable.

He had recently been to have his back brace checked. The orthopedist said not to expect more than a fifty percent correction in the brace. When checked last week, Sam was correcting one hundred percent wearing the brace.

At three months his mother reported general growth. “Even his joints are growing bigger,” she said.

Remember, there is no one homeopathic medicine for dyslexia, for spurring growth, or for scoliosis. Only the medicine that fits the whole person, physically and mentally, can bring about such dramatic changes. When we do find the **most similar** medicine, in this case, *Barya iodatum,* multiple problems can clear up.

eighteen

Conventional Medicine - Multiple Problems, Multiple Drugs / Homeopathy - Multiple Problems - One Medicine

Throughout this book, we have shown how a single homeopathic medicine can often resolve two or more diseases, diseases regarded as distinct and unrelated by conventional medicine. In the following case report, four apparently unrelated medical problems all disappeared with one homeopathic medicine—*Sulphur.*

ROCKY MOUNTAIN SPOTTED FEVER + OPTIC NEURITIS + MUSCULOSKELETAL PAINS + INSOMNIA

A 55 year old woman with Rocky Mountain Spotted Fever (RMSF) sought my help. RMSF is an infectious disease caused by the bacterium, *Rickettsia rickettsii.* It is carried by an infected tick. According to the Center for Disease Control (CDC) the symptoms include fever, nausea, vomiting, muscle pain, headache and lack of appetite. Often there is a rash, abdominal pains, joint pains and diarrhea. Treatment is usually with the antibiotic, doxycycline.

Hers was not a textbook case. A week after the tick bite she experienced sudden light-headedness with profuse sweating. She felt weak and faint. "I thought I was having a heat stroke," she said.

She knew what she was talking about as two years before she had had heat stroke and became weak and faint.

With the RMSF, the following symptoms came on suddenly—head spinning, light-headedness, profuse perspiration and difficulty breathing. She had to lie down and, even then, she felt poorly.

"What would bring on these symptoms?" I asked.

"If I walked 150 feet from the barn to the house, they would come on," she said. After an episode, she had to rest for a day and a half but as soon as she got up the symptoms came back.

She continued to worsen. She lost her appetite, began to vomit and developed sharp pains that wandered from head to foot. She had a mild fever and was confined to bed and was scarcely able to move. She was so sick she could not even get up and go to the doctor. When the fever finally broke and the pains let up a bit, she went to her local doctor who prescribed the antibiotic, doxycycline. She could not tolerate it. Then she took the steroid, prednisone, for five days and the pains went away. When she stopped it, they came back.

She had another problem. When she was 21 years old, in 1975, she began having musculoskeletal pains. These occurred only with the change of seasons. Her medical doctors could find no sign of any of the usual arthritic diseases (rheumatoid arthritis, osteoarthritis, etc.) When winter went to spring, spring to summer, or summer to fall, she experienced terrible pains.

When I asked where, exactly, she felt the pains, she said, "It's like there was something evil between the muscles and the bones—something that did not belong. I would get stiff, creaking joints with bone and muscle pains from head to toe. They'd last anywhere from four days to two or three weeks. If someone touched me, it felt like my whole body would shatter. I'd have a slight temperature and when the fever broke, the pains would leave."

These musculoskeletal pains, that came on only with the change of seasons, had nothing to do with the RMSF. Or did they? Four years ago, she moved to Missouri and the musculoskeletal pains disappeared. But with the RMSF they had returned! So, there was a connection, albeit a mysterious one.

As we continued talking, she mentioned another problem. Seven years ago, she was diagnosed with optic neuritis of the right eye causing pain and blindness in that eye. After a course of the steroid, Solumedrol (methylprednisolone), the vision returned. The pain in the back of that eye, however, was still bothering her. She also had a sleeping problem, falling asleep at 10 p.m., waking at midnight, awake till 4 a.m. and then sleeping until 6 a.m. It had gone on for years.

What, I wondered, could be the connection between that pain and her other problems? For the allopath, there was no connection. The RMSF was infectious; the arthritic pains were inflammatory and without a known cause; the optic neuritis was a neurological inflammation of a specific nerve with no known cause and the sleep disorder had to do with the *reticular formation* in the brainstem–again with no known cause.

She could have sought advice from an infectious disease specialist for the RMSF, a rheumatologist for the musculoskeletal pains, an ophthalmologist for the optic neuritis and a sleep disorder expert for the insomnia. Had she done so, she would have found that each specialist would have prescribed separately with no regard for or interest in what the other specialists were prescribing.

It is characteristic of the specialization of conventional medicine that each specialist regards his area of the body as a kind of fiefdom, an independent domain over which his word is unchallenged. Apparently, the whole patient is of little interest.

ONE ELEPHANT, MANY PARTS

I am reminded of the story, *The Blind Men and the Elephant.* One blind man ran into the elephant's side and declared it a wall; another ran his hand over the tusk and said it was a spear; a third felt of the knee and said it was a tree; a fourth maintained the ear was a fan; a fifth was sure the tail was a rope; and the sixth felt the squirming trunk to be a snake.

Of course, none of the blind men had any conception of the whole elephant.

To continue with my patient: I learned that she had always been sociable and had tended bar for fifteen years. She loved to garden and was handy—could fix most anything. She had artistic talent and did drawing and sewing, albeit more in the past. She was a hard worker and a good money manager. She liked to read "How To" books as well as books on herbal medicine, supplements, etc. "I'm a jack-of-all-trades-master-of-none," she joked.

Her profile fit *Sulphur* because she was sociable, artistic, handy and disliked the heat, being a hot person. She was prescribed a single homeopathic dose of *Sulphur*.

When we spoke three weeks later, she was improving though she was not entirely well. Four weeks after that (seven weeks since the dose of *Sulphur*), she reported, “I feel great. I haven’t felt this good in decades. Nothing hurts. I am also sleeping through the night. It’s been years since I’ve able to do that. And, I no longer have any hot flashes at all.”

I checked my notes. I had no record of hot flashes. Interesting, the correct medicine can cure even those complaints the patient neglects to mention!

“Before your medicine,” she said, “if it was hot outside I couldn’t last in the heat more than two minutes. I’d overheat, sweat and get dizzy.” Now she was tolerating the heat.

“One of the best things,” she added, “is that the pain in the back of the right eye has completely gone! I’ve had it since the optic neuritis was diagnosed seven years ago.”

So there was a connection between the optic neuritis, the generalized, sharp, wandering pains, the hot flashes, the insomnia and the RMSF.

The connection was **Sulphur**. This one medicine cured her not only of the RMSF but all the other problems as well. This kind of a result is not unusual in homeopathy. The body, with its apparently separate ailments, is a unity just as *the elephant with its parts is still all elephant.*

It is typical of homeopaths to investigate all the problems the patient complains of, not simply the one the patient comes in with. We try to be inclusive. We look for a single homeopathic medicine that will cover all of the patient’s complaints.

Caution: *Sulphur* will NOT cure every case of RMSF or hot flashes or optic neuritis. *Sulphur* was HOMEOPATHIC to her symptoms, that is, it matched her symptoms and it matched her personality traits. That is the ONLY reason it acted curatively.

nineteen

Another RMSF Complicated By Lyme Disease

It must be emphasized that homeopaths do not have specific medicines for specific diseases. No matter what the disease is called, no matter the name, we always take a complete history inquiring into every facet of the person's illness and life as we strive to find the **simillimum** or medicine that most closely resembles the patient's symptoms.

I have already reported a case of Rocky Mountain Spotted Fever (RMSF) cured with *Sulphur.* Now I wish to detail another case of RMSF, this one complicated by Lyme Disease (LD).

A thirty-year-old woman developed RMSF followed by LD for which she was treated with partial success with antibiotics. She came to me as she had started to relapse.

Just as RMSF is caused by a bacterium carried by an infected tick, so also is LD. *Borrelia burgdorferi* is the culprit in Lyme and also is carried by an infected tick. It causes fever, headache, fatigue, and a skin rash. It can progress into a debilitating disease affecting the joints, heart and nervous system. It is especially well-known for its arthritic symptoms. It, too, is treated with antibiotics which can be successful especially if started early in the disease. Unfortunately, in many cases of both RMSF and LD, antibiotics fail and the patients suffer terribly with the diseases disabling them.

Though the diagnosis is not always easy, this woman's doctors had done the requisite laboratory tests and declared she had Lyme. The diagnosis, for the homeopath, is interesting, but it really does not help in prescribing. For that, the homeopath has to take a complete case.

This patient, I'll call her Jenny, remembered waking up one day in the summer of 2007 with burning spots, one on the abdomen, one on the upper inner thigh and a third along the bra line. She thought it was ringworm. Later, much later, she reasoned, they must have been caused by a tick bite. More about that later.

After a month the lesions went away but soon after Jenny had her third ectopic pregnancy (when the sperm fertilizes the egg in the fallopian tube) and surgery was performed the end of October, 2007. After the surgery she experienced low energy and trouble sleeping. She was waking unrefreshed. She had been a most active person and volleyball was her passion. By the spring and summer of 2008 volleyball was exhausting her. Any exercise resulted in fatigue lasting two days.

She noticed fullness in the ears and, "a ticking sound in the ears when I swallowed." If ice was dropped into a glass the noise was unbearable yet she could not hear someone close when they spoke. Her muscles began to twitch especially on the left side of the body. Facial acne followed with large pustules on the face and neck. There were two episodes of sudden dizziness and nausea with sweating in August, 2008. She lost feeling in the right arm and eventually was unable to move her right hand. In the summer of that year she developed balance problems. On rising from sitting she felt dizzy, as though she were falling to the left. She was bumping into walls and dropping things. It became difficult to find the right word when speaking.

Jenny was diagnosed with the acute form of RMSF in October, 2008. She recalled the skin lesions in the summer of 2007, and figured they must have been caused by a tick bite. But she could not understand how she could test positive for the acute form of RMSF fifteen months later. The test was repeated and was positive again. A few weeks later she tested positive for LD. It is uncommon to have both diseases at the same time. She was placed on doxycycline for several months and did improve.

In January, 2009 she had another failed pregnancy, this one a miscarriage.

After stopping the antibiotics, Jenny gradually began to relapse. It was then that she sought out homeopathic treatment.

"All my symptoms are starting to come back," she said at our first meeting. "The twitching, the clicking in the ears, the fullness in the ears, the decreased hearing, irritability and lower energy—it's all coming back."

I now knew her diagnoses— RMSF and LD—and I knew the particular symptoms that were bothering her. But that information was not enough for me to prescribe on. I needed to know details about her as a person.

I noticed she spoke rapidly and energetically. Her husband helped. "She is very active," he said. "Focused. Very athletic. Definitely not a couch potato. She used to play volleyball all the time."

In school she did poorly on tests and her academic record was not great. Her thing was sports. Besides volleyball, she did track.

She was punctual. "I like to be five minutes early," she said.

She had struggled with depression since she was married in 2003. She came from a large family and in her marriage she was alone a lot since her husband was away often. Also, they moved five times in four years.

I asked how she was when depressed. "I would just lay around," she said. "Not much motivation." She mentioned how much she had enjoyed being around people before her marriage.

She then made curious statement. "I tell the truth," she said.

"What do you mean you tell the truth?" I asked.

"Well my sister lives with us. We found out she was using drugs. I confronted her about it and told her she needed to tell our parents and she did." Jenny, herself, said she had always been a "goody two-shoes" and "a black and white kind of person."

By this point, I suspected she might need the homeopathic medicine, *Sepia*, so—knowing the symptoms *Sepia* women often have with their periods—I asked about them.

"I have to sit on the toilet, sometimes for hours, because I feel everything is going to fall out," she said.

When a woman says that during their menses she feels as if the uterus is going to fall down and out through the vagina, this is a very strong or confirmatory symptom of *Sepia*—this bearing down sensation during menses.

I asked about her housekeeping. "When I was depressed the house would become a wreck, she said." Then I'd get up and clean the whole house in two hours."

"I bet you cleaned to music," I said.

"Yes. How did you know?"

I knew because that is typical of *Sepia* women (and men). They are always better with activity and vigorous exercise. Often they love to dance and if they can't dance they will boogie around the house when cleaning.

She mentioned how before these two illnesses she often used to run six miles effortlessly. *Sepia* people love activity, the more vigorous the better. If they do not do sports they work hard and fast. They tend to be honest (witness how she confronted her sister about her drug use.) And she had the strong bearing-down sensation during her menstrual period.

One other strong *Sepia* trait: they often become indifferent, even hostile, to loved ones. I asked her how she treated her husband.

She replied, "When I was depressed I told him, 'I don't like you. I don't want to be married to you.'"

I was certain she needed *Sepia* and gave her a dose.

During the follow up visit she was ecstatic. "I'm doing a thousand times better," she said. "I feel I'm a completely different person. I told my husband I felt genuinely happy for the first time in years."

"My female parts aren't as heavy as they used to be. Every time I had a period it felt heavy down there—my uterus and lower intestines. Also my thighs felt heavy. Not now."

She had resumed running and it was not tiring her. Also, she was getting on much better with her husband. She even overheard him say to a friend, "She's a completely different person."

Her acne, however, was considerably worse. In homeopathy, it is important to know what is happening on the road to cure. WE LIKE TO SEE OLD SYMPTOMS RETURN AND ACNE WAS AN OLD SYMPTOM. ALSO, WE LIKE TO SEE LESS IMPORTANT ORGANS AND STRUCTURES BEING AFFECTED AS THE MORE IMPORTANT ONES IMPROVE. AS THE ACNE WAS FAR LESS CRUCIAL TO HER HEALTH THAN THE SYMPTOMS SHE HAD HAD EARLIER WITH THE RMSF AND LD, I ASSURED HER THAT EVERYTHING WAS IN ORDER.

Sulphur cured the first woman with RMSF because she was a *Sulphur* type and *Sepia* cured this woman with both RMSF and LD only because she was a *Sepia* type.

Another person with either RMSF or LD will most likely need still another homeopathic medicine. Homeopathy is very different from conventional medicine in this regard. WE FOCUS ON THE INNATE CHARACTERISTICS OF THE PERSON WHICH ARE PARTICULAR TO HIM OR HER. BY "INNATE" I MEAN THOSE TRAITS THAT AN INDIVIDUAL COMES INTO THIS WORLD WITH. THEY SHINE FORTH CONSISTENTLY THROUGHOUT THE LIFE. SEPIA WOULD NOT BE INDICATED IN A LAZY, SLOTHFUL PERSON WHO MOVED SLOWLY THROUGH LIFE. ALWAYS WE TRY TO MATCH THE HOMEOPATHIC MEDICINE WITH THE PATIENT'S CHARACTERISTIC QUALITIES.

twenty

Another Case of Lyme Solved with Homeopathic Opium

Now that two cases of Rocky Mountain Spotted Fever (one complicated by Lyme Disease) have been presented, let's look at another case of Lyme, this one involving the husband of Jenny in the previous chapter.

In homeopathic prescribing it is often a strange trait or habit that leads us to the correct medicine. Such was the case of a man with Lyme Disease who had virtually no sense of danger even when in a dangerous situation. How his fearlessness lead to the medicine that cured him is the subject of this report.

He was a police officer, thirty-two-years old, who tested positive for LD a month before coming in for homeopathic treatment. As I said before, LD is caused by a bacterium, *Borrelia burgdorferi,* which is transmitted by the bite of an infected tick. It causes fever, headache, fatigue and a skin rash. It can progress into a debilitating disease affecting the joints, heart and nervous system. It is especially well-known for its arthritic symptoms. It is usually treated with antibiotics.

Two years earlier he had been bitten by an insect, unseen by him at the time. Sixteen months later, towards the end of 2008, he noticed fatigue. "I started feeling tired all the time," he said. "It was more than sleepiness—it was a deep fatigue." About the same time he became uncharacteristically irritable. "I was quick to snap at my wife and child—very impatient. At the slightest provocation I would become very angry and argumentative."

He put on weight—from 190 pounds to 210—without dieting.

His stamina declined. Where he had run four to six miles a day, he was now pushing to do one mile.

"My mental acuity is way down," he said.

His wife chimed in. "He was normally very quick. Now he takes longer."

"I used to be a pilot in the Air Force," he said, "and I was always making quick decisions. Now, as a police officer in the squad car I'm much slower on the computer and I'm making mistakes."

He was waking at night with one or the other of the upper extremities "paralyzed." It mostly affected the right upper extremity and had occurred once or twice a month for the past year.

"When I sit on the toilet one or both legs from the thighs down go numb on me," he said. "That happens about once a week."

Before he became sick he got by on five to six hours of sleep a night. Gradually, he began to sleep more and more. One day he slept twenty-one hours.

"One day I kept trying to wake him," said his wife. "I spoke to him again and again and later, when he finally did awaken, he didn't remember anything I had said."

He was very groggy for a good two hours after waking. "I feel like a zombie," he said.

I asked about his interests. "I'm an adrenaline junkie," he joked, and related how he had ridden dirt bikes, high performance street bikes and loved to rappel, a technique whereby the climber descends the face of a cliff by sliding down a rope passed under one thigh, across the body, and over the opposite shoulder. He and a friend once rappelled 300 feet down a mountain face.

"And I love being a police officer," he said.

"How are you in dangerous situations?" I asked.

"I feel relaxed," he said very simply and then related how some time ago he had put his cell phone on the roof of his car and forgotten it was there. He drove off and when he got to an intersection he braked causing the phone to slide forward down the windshield, hood and onto the street. It was a busy intersection and though cars were whizzing by he calmly walked to the phone and picked it up.

"How close were the cars to you?"

"They were going right by within a foot or two of my head."

He got back into the car and remarked to his wife, "I think I'm too comfortable around moving cars."

Indeed, I thought so, too, and began thinking of homeopathic *Opium* which is derived from actual opium. Of course, in the process of converting it into the homeopathic preparation it is diluted so many times that no molecules of the original opium remain.

Opium is a medicine that can be useful when the patient sleeps long and deeply and feels groggy on waking which was certainly true of him. People who need *Opium* are often risk takers and can have no sense of danger in situations where most of us would be terrified.

It also covered his other symptoms—numbness and paralysis of the limbs and his irritability. Because people who need homeopathic *Opium* often have keen senses, I asked about his hearing. He said it was acute.

"And your vision?"

"I'm 20/15 in one eye and 20/17 in the other," he said. Normal is 20/20 so his vision was considerably better than normal.

He received a dose of *Opium* and within a few weeks all symptoms resolved. He related how he and his partner responded to a breaking and entering. When they arrived on the scene the perpetrator was swinging a large, heavy object into a door, trying to break it down. They managed to swiftly cuff the suspect and then call various law enforcement agencies in a few minutes. He did his job thoroughly and efficiently and received a commendation from his senior officer.

Obviously, his mental acuity was better than ever. He has remained well.

The conventional treatment for LD is to take antibiotics for weeks, sometimes months, and even with the treatment many patients fail to recover. This man recovered with one dose of high potency *Opium*.

As I report these cases, homeopathy must seem stranger and stranger. One case of RMSF cured with *Sulphur*, another RMSF complicated by LD cured with *Sepia*, and a case of LD cured with *Opium*. And in every case almost no attention paid to the complaint the patient came in with!

In the next two chapters we'll look at other cases of *Opium*. Though the patients' problems are not at all similar, the underlying *Opium* theme will be present.

twenty one

Another Opium Case: Concussion

In case after case, one sees that homeopaths literally do NOT treat the disease of the person but rather the person with the disease. In this third case of homeopathic *Opium*, it proved helpful after a head injury.

Let's entertain, for a moment, the idea that illness 'perambulates,' that is, it moves about, strolls, and roams around the mind/body complex. I want to convey the idea that illness or disease or sickness is rarely fixed to one organ or one system. Instead, symptoms appear here and there in an apparently unrelated manner.

A twelve-year-old boy was brought in by his parents the end of March, 2011. When I asked why he had come, he said, "My stomach has been hurting a lot for two weeks."

"How does it feel?" I asked.

"It feels like I'm being stabbed with a knife."

On questioning, it turned out the "stomach" pain was actually in the left upper quadrant of the abdomen.

His parents chimed in. "He had a concussion in November of last year."

"How did it happen?"

"I was wrestling and got thrown."

"Did you lose consciousness?" I asked. Head injuries commonly come on after a loss of consciousness.

"No. But my Dad said I needed help walking."

"At first, his right pupil responded to light slower than the left," his father said, "and his eyes were glassy. He became unusually sensitive to noise."

"He was slow to respond to questions," his mother added.

He improved slowly. Even now, four months later, he was not back to normal. An electroencephalogram was normal. No MRI was done. A cognitive test, done in early December, was abnormal. Later ones showed significant improvement but the family was told he would probably not be back to normal until the summer of 2011.

Since the concussion, he found it harder to concentrate. Before, he took few notes in class and simply listened. That was enough to do okay on tests. Since the injury, he found it harder to absorb what was being said.

"I am less energetic," he said. "Also, I'm irritable."

His mother said, "He has fairly good energy until about 6 p.m. Then his energy plummets. At 9 p.m. he can no longer stay up. And he wakes tired at 6:30 a.m."

At this point in the interview, most of the findings were expected, that is to say, they were common in patients with concussions. Mild cognitive impairment, low energy, waking tired, irritability and sensitivity to noise are all associated with concussions. But the stabbing pain in the left upper quadrant didn't compute. It was anomalous, that is, it really didn't fit in with the usual presentation of a concussion. The anomalous always is of interest to the homeopath. The problem was: how to include it. At this point I did not have enough to prescribe on.

I asked about his sleep and was told it was deep and always had been. Also, I learned that if he lost sleep, the following day was considerably harder.

In addition, he was hot-natured (good body heat, disliked hot weather) and was thirsty for cold water.

Why is it important if the patient is hot or cold? It turns out that our medicines, in their provings, tended to make the provers feel either hotter or colder than they usually felt. So, when choosing a medicine, we try to choose a "hot" medicine for a hot-natured person and a "cold" medicine for a cold-natured person. The medicine selected should correspond, as nearly as possible, to the patient.

At this point, I was thinking of homeopathic *Opium*. It is listed under "Head, injuries of the head; after:" but *Opium* is one of forty-three medicines in that rubric. So, I had to distinguish *Opium* from forty-two other medicines known to help head injuries. What is characteristic of those who need *Opium* is that they tend to be befuddled and have poor concentration. Many of those who benefit from *Opium* sleep very deeply (remember the policeman?). They are usually hot-natured. Also, they are often surprisingly indifferent to pain.

"How do you react to a fall, a scrape, an injury? Is it fairly painful or not particularly so?"

"Oh, I usually just get up and keep on," he said. In the Repertory, is the rubric, "Painlessness of symptoms usually painful," and there is *Opium.*

I was now satisfied that his **state** corresponded to *Opium,* and he was given a single dose of the one-thousandth potency, i.e., diluted one thousand times, each time one to one hundred.

When seen three weeks later, I learned that he improved within twenty-four hours. At the follow up he said, "I felt clearer in my head after I started the medicine. I have no more stomach pain." The left upper quadrant pain, his mother said, vanished the first day after the *Opium* not to return. He now had no energy dip at 6 p.m. and was able to stay up till 10 to 10:30 p.m. with decent energy. He was concentrating better at school and absorbing the material more easily. His father noted, "Since your medicine, he gives more in depth, nuanced responses when we speak."

He still tired a bit quickly on playing basketball, but he was definitely ninety percent improved. No more medicine given.

Though it is hard to understand how the abdominal pain could be related to the concussion, the fact it disappeared with *Opium* at the same time that his cognition and energy improved suggests they were related.

How does one know if the *Opium* acted? Many mild head injury patients do slowly improve on their own. In this case, the improvement was swift–overnight. All parameters improved right away, including the abdominal pain suggesting *Opium* acted globally, i.e., on mind and body at once.

Materia Medica Pura contains Hahnemann's original provings of many important medicines of his time. The chapter on *Opium* contains not only proving symptoms but many, many reports of eating or smoking opium which Hahnemann gathered from the existing medical literature on opium. He always referred to these scholars as "old school authorities" and every symptom he included in *Materia Medica Pura* that came from one of them he carefully referenced. Hahnemann always maintained that toxicological reports of the gross substances were as valid as the proving symptoms that resulted from using the potentized substances. All Hahnemann's many provings contained both kinds of data.

From his study of the literature on opium and from his proving of *Opium*, Hahnemann concluded that the drug had a primary action and a secondary action. Primary actions, mostly short-lived, can be extreme contentedness, tranquility, delightful fantasies, cheerfulness, high-spirits, courageous to the point of rashness, and heightening of the senses.

Some primary actions of opium from *Materia Medica Pura*:

- Cheerfulness, liveliness, contentment, increased strength.
- Courage, intrepidity, magnanimity.
- Intrepidity in danger.
- Daring wildness.

Several of these *Opium* symptoms were used in the case of the policeman. Other symptoms of regular opium that the policeman and the boy with the concussion had:

- Great inclination to sleep.
- The sleep caused by opium passed into an unusual stupefaction.

Some secondary actions of *Opium* from *Hahnemann's Materia Medica Pura*:

- Increases the heat of the whole body and leaves dryness of the mouth and thirst.
- Unconquerable lassitude.
- Cloudiness of the head.
- Dullness in the head.

- Stupefaction of the intellect.
- Stupefaction and insensibility.
- Obtuseness of the intellect.
- Indifference to pain and pleasure.
- She knew not what was going on around her and gave no sign of feeling.

In the introductory section on *Opium* in *Materia Medica Pura* Hahnemann writes:

> The oriental indulgers in opium, after sleeping off their opium intoxication, are always in a state of secondary opium action; their mental faculties are much weakened by too frequent indulgence in the drug. Chilly, pale, bloated, trembling, spiritless, weak, stupid, and with a perceptible anxious inward malaise, they stagger in the morning into the tavern to take their allowance of opium pills in order to quicken the circulation of their blood and obtain warmth, to revive their depressed vital spirits, to reanimate their dulled fantasy with some ideas, and to infuse, in a palliative way, some activity into their paralyzed muscles.

To recap: homeopathic *Opium* can have two fairly distinct presentations:

1. The super alive, courageous, risk taker with acute hearing and vision. May be a light sleeper but not always.
2. The dull, indifferent, dopey, sleepyhead. Usually is a deep sleeper. This situation may have come on from a strong fright.

Both *Opium* types often have high pain thresholds. In practice, one sees mostly the first *Opium* type or the second. Sometimes, however, the patient needing *Opium* can have a mix of symptoms.

Opium is an indispensable homeopathic medicine and NEVER has any of the deleterious effects of the drug, opium.

twenty two

More Opium: The Zombie

Having reported on the policeman with Lyme Disease and the twelve year old with a head injury, both helped substantially with homeopathic *Opium*, I now report on an apparently "depressed" young woman, whose life was dramatically and permanently changed with *Opium*.

Perhaps no medicine in our homeopathic materia medica has more apparently contradictory symptoms than *Opium*. The case report that follows is about a young woman who could not have been more different from the police officer yet *Opium* changed her life.

This nineteen-year-old gave the impression of someone who was scarcely present. She appeared detached, vague, disinterested. The word "zombie" came to mind. One definition of zombie is a dead body that has been brought back to life. Another definition—someone who acts or responds like an automaton, i.e., in a mechanical or apathetic way. She seemed to fit both definitions.

Her mother said, "She has poor motivation. She becomes confused if she has decisions to make."

I saw her in January, 1996. She had been on anti-depressants twice, once in 1989, again toward the end of 1994.

At one point, she moved out of her mother's house to live with her father. The parents were divorced. For an entire year she hardly left her bedroom. I asked her why.

"When I'm depressed, I want to hide," she said.

"Her way to handle things is not to speak, to be passive, to withdraw," said her mother.

There was a time when her weight went from 130 lbs. to 98 lbs. yet, she maintained, she was unaware of the weight loss. That surprised me. How could a teenaged girl not be aware of a 32 lb. weight loss?

I asked if she were depressed now. She said she was not, but her manner, expression and posture suggested otherwise.

When she did become angry with someone, she would simply stop talking to that person, cut them off for months at a time. She was known in the family to be malicious.

When she was five years old, her parents divorced. Her mother had been married a total of four times.

"How do you feel about the fact your mother has had four marriages?"

"I don't feel any resentment against my parents."

I was beginning to think she didn't feel much of anything, resentment included.

"Last year I got depressed and didn't notice it," she said. "By the time we noticed it, I couldn't get out of bed."

During that depression, she lived on a ranch and slept a lot and played with her dogs. The dogs helped. She said she loved animals and preferred them to people. Mostly though, she wanted to be alone.

Her mother spoke of her good qualities. "She is dependable and responsible. She is punctual. She saves her money. But I don't think she is equipped to take care of herself."

The girl said she did not know why she had no motivation. The very idea of choosing a career and making important life choices was "overwhelming."

When she had a busy day with lots of activities, she felt better. "I work well under pressure," she said.

She constantly felt overheated. "I use the air conditioning in the car in the winter," she said. Hot, stuffy rooms were unbearable. She sought cool places.

Asked what was most important in her life, she said, "I haven't stopped to think about that. I don't have any idea. I guess I want everything to be calm and organized and not rushed. I want stability." She disliked being pressured to make decisions.

Her mother recalled that at six weeks of age, she had pneumonia. "She never fussed or complained with that pneumonia," said her mother. "Another thing, she never complained about any of my marriages or divorces."

Her indifference extended to the physical. Once a horse broke a post. It went flying and struck her. She never complained! She and her mother agreed that she never got upset about anything.

When she was a small child she used to disappear into her room around 8:30 p.m. every night. She never asked her mother for help with homework and never asked for money.

Her indifference extended to food though she admitted to eating mostly junk food.

Her level of disinterest was appalling. She had been vegetating—doing nothing—most of her life. She seemed literally not to care about anything. Clearly, she had been, and probably still was, depressed. But it was deeper than that. It was a profound **apathy**.

There were two striking physical symptoms: she was hot-natured and had a high threshold to physical pain.

This young woman gave the impression of being scarcely alive. Nothing seemed to affect her, not her mother's four divorces, not her pneumonia at age six weeks, not being struck by a flying post.

She didn't care if her mother helped her with her homework or not; she did not notice a 32 lb. weight loss; she never asked for money.

I consulted my repertory and used the following rubrics (symptoms):

- Indifference, does not complain + Complaining, never.
- Indifference – joyless.
- Unfeeling.
- Asking for nothing.
- Senses - dull.
- Painlessness of complaints usually painful.
- Warmth aggravates.

Running through all the rubrics was homeopathic *Opium*. I chose it because one of the effects of smoking opium is to depress the sensorium—those areas of the brain that process and register incoming sensory information and make possible the conscious awareness of the world. Her conscious awareness of the world was dimmed—drastically so.

She received a single dose of homeopathic *Opium* which, as mentioned earlier, contained no molecules of regular opium.

When I saw her six weeks later, she was a different person.

"I have been working for the IRS for the last three weeks and I'm enjoying it," she announced.

A year ago at this time, she had been depressed, unable to concentrate and cried a lot. "Now I look forward to going to work. I'm planning to do a degree in the fall. I haven't felt this good in I don't know how long. I used to feel hopeless. Now I'm looking forward to life."

Asked when was the last time she felt this good, she said, "I don't ever remember feeling this good. I feel my entire life I've been in a shell."

We spoke more about how she had been prior to *Opium.* She remembered that when she had been depressed she would wake frequently "every hour on the hour." She had never slept deeply and had never slept through an alarm or telephone. People who need *Opium* often sleep as though drugged, not hearing alarms, even thunder, but others who need *Opium* sleep lightly. She was one of the latter. She remembered how even in the fourth grade she would wake up every hour all night long. "And you know, it was just like when I was depressed later on. I never wanted to talk to anyone then and for most of my life."

I said, "You know, I thought you were depressed when I first met you six weeks ago but you said you weren't. Was I mistaken?"

"No, she said, "You were right. I was depressed." She went on, "I've never felt good my whole life. I don't feel like myself anymore. I feel like a new person."

She was less bothered by the heat and had even been wearing a sweater to work. With the correct homeopathic medicine overly hot people become less hot and overly chilly people become less chilly.

We talked about her response to pain and I learned that throughout her life, even as a child, she never noticed pain. "I never cried. I was never scared when other kids were." Once, she was hit by a board in the back of her head and her vision blurred. She was unable to see for a few seconds. "I don't remember it hurting at all." She was taken to the ER and a hairline fracture was found!

"As a child, I remember just sitting and watching, watching the world go by. I was never part of it."

One week after the *Opium*, she announced to her mother, "I feel well," and started to look for a house. "I feel I have a whole new life ahead of me."

Her mother talked more about her pneumonia when she was a baby. "I stayed up with her night and day. I was afraid she was going to die. You know, she never cried."

As we continued to talk, more and more fascinating details of her life emerged. Her mother spoke of giving birth and how she rushed to get to the hospital, driving at high speed. She arrived at 3 a.m. The child was born ten minutes later. "I was scared," said her mother. I was afraid I'd have the baby in the car. The nurses made me go to the bathroom. I was terrified I'd have the baby in the toilet. They insisted I get up and walk to the table. They said I'd have to wait for the doctor. They said, 'You've got to wait till the doctor gets here.' It turned out the doctor was on his way to the racetrack. I was scared. I loved my doctor and he promised me he'd be there.

"I told the nurses I was having a baby and they said I couldn't be as I wasn't dilated. But that happened to me the first time (first birth) and the same thing happened to my mother."

The mother's story of the birth confirmed my theory. She came into this world the product of a great fright on the part of her mother. Smoking opium is known to cause fright in some users. Somehow, her mother's fright imprinted itself onto her whole being—mind and body—making her insensible not only to pain but insensible to all of life. The product of a shock, she turned into a zombie. *Opium* broke the spell and returned her to life. Of course, her mother was NOT similarly affected. She processed the fright and carried on. Her daughter, with her delicate new brain and highly sensitive nervous system, kept the imprint of the fright for nineteen years.

I did not see her for years but her mother reported she was doing well, that she had married and had a child.

On June 5, 2007, she brought her son in for treatment. Asked how she had been, she said the nineteen year depression had never returned.

twenty three

How A Poisonous Snake Venom Can Be Curative - A Case Of Eczema Followed By Severe Anxiety - The Need For Two Medicines

Most case histories presented thus far show a single homeopathic medicine making a significant improvement in the health of the patient. It is ideal when a single medicine works deeply and resolves one or more problems. But it is not always so. People often have complex problems and sometimes need more than one medicine to get well. The classical homeopath does not combine medicines, but may have to change medicines in the course of treatment which may extend over months, even years.

Farok was such a patient. I saw him in March, 2010. He was thirty-one, married with two small children and held a job editing books on science. He lived in Vermont. He came for eczema of his left leg which was swollen, reddish-blue with a tinge of purple and crusty. It had recently begun to move to the right leg but the lesion there was far less extensive. There was mild eczema on the arms.

In 2002, he fractured two bones in the left foot and sprained the left knee. He was prescribed an orthopedic boot in lieu of a cast. After some time wearing the boot, the left leg became hot and painful. The diagnosis: a clot in one of the deep veins of the leg known as Deep Vein Thrombosis (DVT). It is considered a semi-emergency because such clots can break free of the wall of the vein and travel upward, through the heart and into the pulmonary artery. Such a clot is known as a pulmonary embolism. If large enough, it can infarct the lungs causing widespread necrosis in the lung, even death. He was therefore hospitalized and given IV heparin, an anticoagulant. When discharged, heparin was stopped and he was placed on an oral anticoagulant, coumadin, for six months. All DVTs are treated in this manner. He recovered nicely from the DVT and the fractures healed, but the left leg remained swollen. It was there the eczema appeared. Of late, it had begun to move to the right leg. Often a skin lesion or an arthritic condition will localize to one side of the body and sometimes, as in this man, it will start on one side and move to the other. His was a stubborn eczema.

An apparently unrelated problem: he sometimes stumbled and bumped into furniture and walls.

As you now know, the homeopath pays more attention to the person than to the illness. Farok disliked the cold yet preferred cold drinks. In fact, he chewed ice daily. It turned out his thirst was not for water but beer. He was drinking twelve a day and had a history of drug abuse. In his late teens, he abused many drugs. He recounted the time he boiled a *Datura stramonium* plant and drank a glass. *D. stramonium* contains *hyoscine*, as well as *atropine*, *hyoscyamine*, *apohyoscine*, and *meteloidine* making it poisonous as well as hallucinogenic.

He recalled his experience: "I saw things crawling over my skin–black dots. I saw a baby lying in bed. The TV turned into my friend and we'd talk. I fell to my knees in front of the TV talking to it. I loved the visuals-the feel of it. I liked the distortions of reality."

At age twenty-one his parents had him admitted to a detox facility in Minnesota where he spent some weeks. It helped, temporarily, but he continued to use.

When I saw him he was occasionally smoking Wild Lettuce (*Lactuca virosa*) which has mild hallucinogenic properties as well as marijuana and K-2, synthetic cannabis.

Strangely, he had been a model child who was entirely truthful, always went to school, studied before he would go out to play. Adults thought of him as unusually mature. That all changed in his teenage years when he went heavily into dope. He admitted he was now on the lazy side.

His adventures as an addict, though interesting, could not lead to a successful homeopathic prescription. For that, I needed to know those features that could not be explained by either drug use or the fact he had eczema.

As the homeopath is taking the history, he is a bit like a detective looking for an outstanding clue which will enable him to crack the case. We call it an **entry point**. For me, the entry point was that he was chilly **and** liked to eat ice. I consulted my repertory. There are relatively few homeopathic medicines known to produce a desire for ice. With a few more questions, I discovered he disliked tight clothes including shoes, socks, neckties and belts. Intolerance of snug clothing is a strong characteristic of all snake medicines. I needed a "cold" snake medicine and *Elaps corallinus*, the Coral Snake, fit the description. Quickly reading up on *Elaps* I learned that *Elaps*, in its proving, caused an increase in ear wax.

"What is your ear wax like?" I wanted to know.

"I have a lot of ear wax," he replied. A point for *Elaps.*

I continued reading about *Elaps* and learned people needing *Elaps* tended to bite, not their nails, but their fingers. "Do you bite your fingers?" I asked.

He held up his fingers. They were lined with cut marks, some bloody, some healing. Another point for *Elaps.*

I took the following symptoms:

- The skin lesion moving from the left leg to the right.
- Cold-natured (could not bear cold weather).
- Desire for ice.
- Increased earwax.
- Biting fingers.
- Laziness

These were a strange group of symptoms to link up in one person. Even stranger, they are all found in the homeopathic medicine, *Elaps corallinus*, the Brazilian Coral Snake. Homeopaths would say that Farok was in a state of *Elaps*, i.e., he needed *Elaps* because *Elaps* can cause and cure those symptoms. I knew then I would give him *Elaps.* But first, I asked him how he reacted to snakes.

"My dog got bit by a snake on her throat," he said. "I sucked the venom out. That night I saw shapes, cubes, squares."

As all signs and symptoms pointed to *Elaps*, he was given a single dose.

At the one month follow up, the eczema had gone from the arms, a very good sign as we like to see skin lesions improve from the top of the body first and later from the lower parts. It had also disappeared from the right leg. Remember, it had started on the left leg and moved to the right. We also like to see improvement in the reverse order of occurrence, so this was another good sign (Chapter Fifty).

It is worth emphasizing that homeopaths pay a lot of attention to laterality, that is, the side of the body the symptoms appear on. In Farok's case, he had fractured two bones in the left foot, sprained the left knee and suffered a DVT in the left leg and then, finally, developed eczema on the left leg. Accordingly, we wanted a homeopathic medicine that mostly affects the left side. *Elaps* not only affects the left side but is also known to heal problems that begin on the left and extend to the right, exactly as his eczema had.

He was now drinking half as many beers. He was still biting his fingers but was no longer running into walls or stumbling.

Two months later, he said, "My eczema is almost completely gone. My left leg is a white-pink and still swollen. There is no itching."

He was still biting his fingers. Not running into walls or stumbling. He was using marijuana once a day and drinking six to twelve beers a day.

After another month, he said of the skin condition, "It is almost gone." But he was biting his hands more and drinking twelve beers a day. Not using marijuana. Three weeks earlier, his blood pressure had spiked giving him a scare. "I thought I was having a heart attack," he said. "Or it might have been a panic attack." He went back on his blood pressure medicines. A cardiologist did a stress test which was normal as were the heart enzymes.

How to evaluate Farok? He came to homeopathy for eczema and it was virtually gone. Gone, too, was the ataxia (inability to coordinate muscular movement). His tendency to drink too much had not budged and he was still biting his fingers and hands. He was pleased. I was not. I did not like the fact his blood pressure was not controlled nor was I pleased he was still biting his hands, a deep-seated nervous habit.

I did not talk to Farok for another fifteen months. When I did, he was beside himself with anxiety. "I've been feeling anxious for months," he said. He spoke of being jealous of his wife. "It's irrational. She's never given me cause. But I have panic attacks thinking I'll lose her."

I asked about the eczema. "It is gone," he said. "The leg is still discolored and swollen but there is no itching. It's pretty normal."

He quit all alcohol for four months, April through July, then started in again. "I did a lot of cocaine in September," he said, then started talking again about the jealousy. "I've always been a jealous person. I ruined a relationship ten years ago. I was suspicious when I should not have been."

He said he was still biting his fingers, "but a lot less." He was no longer eating ice, but still liked cold drinks. He remained on the chilly side. His nerves couldn't bear the screaming of children (he had two small ones at home).

He then described how uncomfortable he became when he went into a public place. "When I am in a mall, I feel embarrassed. I think people are seeing me, that they are thinking unfavorable thoughts about me."

This last comment astounded me. Farok was volunteering a keynote symptom of *Calcarea carbonica*, namely, a fear of being observed. I quickly asked him a few questions to confirm *Calcarea carbonica* and learned he had a strong fear of heights and that he worried about his health. "If I have a cut, I'll think I have AIDS," he said. People who need *Calcarea* tend to be cold yet like cold drinks, have a fear of heights, worry unduly about their health and hate to be the center of attention. Farok received a single dose of *Calcarea carbonica* and when I talked to him a month later he was much better.

"Five days after starting the medicine," he said, "I felt a lot better. The jealous feelings are pretty much gone. The children screaming doesn't bother me so much and I no longer feel the need to control my wife or kids. Before, it was pretty bad."

As to his anxiety, he said, "I have barely any anxiety at all."

"How about going to the mall?"

"Absolutely no nervousness when I go to a store or mall."

"How do you feel in a crowd?"

"All that is gone," he said. "I have no thoughts that people are looking at me or thinking funny thoughts about me."

Farok was still drinking six beers a day. "It's more than I'd like to," he said. He was still biting his fingers.

Was Farok cured? No, but, clearly, he was much improved. I spoke to his wife. "He's so much better," she said. "The whole house is happier."

He still bit his fingers and there was no guarantee he wouldn't use drugs again and he drank a lot of beer. Cured? It depends on how one looks at cure. George Vithoulkas, a famous Greek homeopath, once suggested that sickness and disease limit one both physically and mentally. As one improves, one becomes less limited and freer to enjoy one's life.

Elaps carollinus had removed the eczema and, much later, *Calcarea carbonica* had removed his anxiety. Farok definitely had more freedom to enjoy his life.

* About one year ago, he stopped all alcohol and recreational drugs.

twenty four

I have been presenting case after case where the correct homeopathic medicine caused dramatic improvements, sometimes on many levels. The real trick to getting good results in homeopathy is in the interview. We call it, "Taking the case." It's not so easy.

PITFALLS IN CASE TAKING. HOW TO BE OBJECTIVE

The initial visit with a homeopath largely consists of an in-depth interview with the patient during which we observe carefully and listen even more carefully. We may also do a physical examination though the physical examination, while important, often does not produce as many clues as do the listening and observing. When the patient cannot speak for himself as in the case of comatose patients, small infants, and patients with speech impediments due to a neurological condition such as a stroke, we then interview someone who knows the patient well. Usually it is a family member or a close friend.

Sometimes, the patient, himself, is a liar and we may be fooled. In such cases, it helps to have another person present to let us know about the lying habit. Sometimes, the patient is delirious or mad and getting to the essential information can be daunting.

Despite an initial interview lasting an hour and a half or longer, we don't always find the curative medicine the first time round. There are a number of reasons for this. Sometimes, the patient fails to mention an important piece of information. Perhaps he forgot; perhaps he considered it unimportant. Sometimes, the homeopath fails to ask pertinent questions, i.e., those questions that elicit crucial information.

For most homeopaths, the main problem in taking a good case is the homeopath himself. What happens in homeopathy, as in all problem solving activities, is the human mind tends to seize an interesting bit of information, decide it is important and follows **it** rather than carefully putting that information to one side and continuing to gather information. The homeopath, like the lazy detective, has to rein himself in from concluding too quickly. Just because the gun that killed the person is in that person's hand does not rule out a homicide.

Hahnemann was well aware of this problem. In the *Organon*, paragraph 83, he writes:

> The individualizing examination of a case of disease…demands of the physician nothing but freedom from prejudice and sound senses, attention in observing and fidelity in tracing the picture of the disease.

Our problem is that it is extraordinarily difficult to keep the mind free of prejudice. Suppose the patient is obese and the homeopath thinks to himself, "With some will power, she wouldn't eat so much. With some will power, she'd exercise more."

Suppose the homeopath is Caucasian and his patient is black and does not speak standard English. The homeopath thinks, "This is a lower class person. Can't even speak correctly."

Suppose the patient is pregnant and unmarried and the homeopath is a strict Christian and is uncomfortable with out of wedlock pregnancies. Suppose the patient is from India and her English is somewhat unclear and the homeopath learns she has been in the United States for thirty years and still has not learned English well. He thinks, "She is a lazy person."

Suppose the homeopath is male and highly sexed and his patient is female and quite attractive and he becomes aroused. How will he maintain his objectivity?

Examples abound. The point is–it is difficult, if not impossible, to maintain an attitude free of prejudice.

The problem of prejudice, unfortunately, is hydra-headed. Every homeopath knows a few key symptoms associated with every major homeopathic medicine. These are known as **keynote** symptoms. All homeopaths know that people needing *Sulphur* are hot, uncover their feet in bed, like to philosophize and are usually sociable types. Let's say the homeopath learns his patient is hot and uncovers his feet in bed. He then seizes on those symptoms and systematically tries to elicit other symptoms characteristic of *Sulphur.* This can prove to be a huge mistake for there are several thousand other symptoms of Sulphur and there are other hot-natured medicines that also uncover their feet in bed.

Similarly with *Pulsatilla.* It is well-known *Pulsatilla* types are hot-natured, thirstless and mild-mannered. The homeopath determines his patient is hot, thirstless and mild, and he is off to the races. Rather than carefully continuing to take a complete history he spends the rest of the hour trying to confirm that his patient needs *Pulsatilla.* Sure of his facts, he gives *Pulsatilla* and then is surprised a month later at the follow up to learn *Pulsatilla* has failed.

Or, let's say the homeopath has learned that people needing *Phosphorus* have left-sided symptoms, are chilly, like consolation and enjoy being with people. He has such a patient in front of him except that his patient prefers to be alone. He therefore rules out *Phosphorus* because he is ignorant that a minority of *Phosphorus* patients do not like company and prefer to be alone. *Phosphorus* is thereby missed and the patient does not get well.

Another example: the patient feels bruised and sore all over. Normally, this would lead the homeopath to think of *Arnica.* But *Arnica* patients invariably feel sore and bruised after an accident or sports injury. The person in front of him feels sore and bruised but reports no history of trauma. *Arnica* is therefore discarded yet the patient, indeed, needs *Arnica.* See the *Arnica* case in which the patient did beautifully on *Arnica* though there was no history of physical trauma (Chapter Fourteen).

The point is that pitfalls abound when taking a case. The homeopath may have prejudices concerning his patient which he may not be aware of or only dimly aware of yet they affect his ability to "see" and understand his patient. He may unwittingly overvalue one or two keynote symptoms and fail to take a complete history. He concludes, erroneously, that the patient needs such and such a medicine and, of course, that medicine fails.

Homeopathy is a difficult art and the best of us can fail.

If one can **not** rush to judgment and simply follow the symptoms and see where they lead, the result can be surprising. In the following case, I allowed the symptoms to speak for themselves and was amazed at the medicine that appeared in the repertorization.

The patient was a sixty-year-old man, formerly in the merchant marine, who had been my patient for about five years. As long as I had known him, he was always hearty, jovial, and intensely alive. On this day he had come in with his wife and, after I finished taking her case, he asked her to leave and then shut the door.

He started out with physical problems. "It is hard to open my eyes in the morning," he said. "It's been going on for the last two or three months. I have coarse grains in my eyes. When I open my eyes I see zigzags. They are like lightning. Also, for the last three or four weeks I have a strong itch in the anus. I last had it twelve years ago."

He had been under quite a lot of stress in the past year. He was operated on for prostate cancer and had recovered nicely. That was followed by a painful attack of herpes zoster, also known as shingles. His mother was dying in another country and that was a constant stress.

But what came next shocked me. In a level voice he said, "The reason I asked my wife to leave is that I don't want her to hear what I have to say. I have a sense of doom—that my life is finished, that I'm going to die soon. The life of the captain is over." He spoke calmly, matter-of-factly.

I was shocked. It was so unlike him. He had always been a robust person with a ready smile and joke. And now this!

"When did this start?"

"A few weeks back, after I came back here after visiting my mother in Europe." He continued, "I know I am unhappy that she is dying," he said almost as an afterthought. He then mentioned that he was having trouble with one of his sons. "He treats me with disrespect," he said. "Also, my two sisters who are looking after our mother don't treat me very well."

He related a dream. "I saw three, maybe four, people enclosed in wall. The wall is covered in glass. I know they will be there forever."

To me, neither the fact of his mother dying or his family not treating him well could explain his conviction that his life was finished. It was beyond explanation. **At this point we come to the beauty of homeopathy. We don't need an explanation. We simply take each symptom at face value, combine them into a totality of the symptoms and see where they point.**

I took the following symptoms from the repertory:

- Vision–zigzags.
- Eye–agglutinated in the morning.
- Eye–opening the lids difficult.
- Mind–death, conviction of.
- Mind–delusions, die, time has come to.
- Mind–delusions, appreciated, he is not.
- Mind–delusions, he cannot exist any longer.
- Mind–delusions, about to die.

Those symptoms yielded *Thuja occidentalis.*

Thuja also has the twin delusions: 1) that he is fragile, and 2) that he is made of glass which reminded me of his dream of people being enclosed in glass. Though I found the dream interesting, I did not include it in the repertorization.

After thirty some years of studying homeopathy and using it to treat thousands of patients, I had no idea that *Thuja* had, in its pathogenesis, such mental symptoms. But there they were. A single dose in the 200c potency cured his eye problem and his mental state and when I saw him six weeks later he was his old jovial self. His mental state lifted immediately; the eye symptoms went away gradually.

Only by leaving aside all my preconceived notions of how *Thuja* was **supposed** to present (based on reading various authors of materia medica and case studies by modern homeopaths) was I able to let the symptoms "fall where they may." In the process I learned that *Thuja occidentalis* can be useful not only in chronic illness but also acute mental states. I also learned to trust the "Totality of the symptoms."

twenty five

Paranoia and Allergies

If one were to ask, "What is the relation between seasonal allergies and paranoia?" the answer would be, "There is none."

And that is correct...much of the time. However, I once treated a young man with seasonal allergies who, I learned, was packing a pistol and was, indeed, paranoid, not paranoid crazy, but consumed with ideas that he was under potential attack, that there were bad people out there out to get him.

I first saw him in 1997 when he was twenty-nine years old. He came in for moderately severe allergies, worse in the spring and summer. The allergy symptoms were the usual: itchy nose, palate, eyes and Eustachian tubes, plus sneezing and occasional loss of smell. Such symptoms homeopaths call "common symptoms" and it is virtually impossible to prescribe successfully on common symptoms as all seasonal allergy sufferers describe the same symptoms. Unlike conventional medicine where antihistamine will grant temporary relief, there is no single medicine in homeopathy for allergies. Every homeopathic patient will need a different medicine based on his or her individuality.

By now, you realize that the homeopath does not target the disease directly, but attempts to learn all he can about his patient in an effort to treat all aspects of the person.

On the physical level, I learned the sweat on his feet was irritating and offensive and was causing the skin to harden and later peel off. "I have to peel off my socks at the end of the day," he said. "It is uncomfortable to walk." This information would turn out to be more relevant in selecting his homeopathic medicine than any of his allergy symptoms.

His gums tended to bleed, again, a fairly common symptom. He was intolerant to cow's milk, an extremely common symptom.

His manner was friendly and open. He admitted being somewhat fearful when alone. "I need people around me," he said.

He then mentioned that he had a permit to carry a handgun and always carried one. "We're a hated group," he said.

"Who is hated?" I wanted to know.

"The government. You always have to watch your back."

He worked at the Houston Intercontinental Airport for the U.S. Immigration and Customs Enforcement. The work was stressful, up to ten to twelve hours a day, sometimes for fourteen days in a row. He allowed or disallowed entry to passengers from abroad. He needed a certain level of awareness and discernment in order to spot illegals. As he spoke Spanish fluently, he often dealt with Central and South Americans.

He went on about how he felt. "I've always been suspicious of people since I was a kid," he said. "I've always had a backup plan. Especially in relationships. When I had a girlfriend, I dated on the side."

"Why?"

"Fear I'll be hurt by her, that she'll take my trust and break it."

His suspiciousness extended beyond personal relationships. "I keep my guard up," he said. "Everyday I use strategies to find out if people are on the up and up. Yet I can be a very deceitful and conniving person myself. Life is a chess game. If you let people take advantage of you, they will."

Because of his hyper vigilance and mistrustfulness, I searched the repertory for clues and found these two rubrics: "Delusion, everyone is an enemy," and "Delusion, he is surrounded by enemies." In both rubrics are found homeopathic mercury known to homeopaths as *Mercurius solubilis. Mercurius* also covers painful peeling of the soles of the feet and bleeding gums. Though most of his allergy symptoms were common, he had one that was strange: he sneezed when he went into bright sunlight. That was an anomaly, something not expected in allergy and it was a symptom of *Mercurius sulphuricum*, an analog of *Mercurius.*

People who need *Mercurius* are often suspicious and mistrustful. When these traits become entwined with anger, *Mercurius* people can be capable of extreme violence, including homicide. Fortunately, my patient was a long way from that.

He received a single dose of *Mercurius sulphuricum* in May, 1997.

Four weeks later, he reported the skin on the soles was no longer hard, the foot sweat no longer irritating or offensive, and the gums had stopped bleeding. The allergies had improved then returned a week ago so he took one dose of *Arundo*, a homeopathic medicine which is known to act in allergies. It helped though I was not pleased he had taken it as I wanted the deeper acting medicine, *Mercurius sulphuricum*, to take care of everything. I was not to be disappointed.

Four months later, in October, the allergies were back and the skin on the soles was becoming harder. *Mercurius sulphuricum* was repeated for the second time.

In May, 1998, he reported he had been fine until the end of February when the allergies returned. "I no longer carry a handgun wherever I go," he said, "though I carry one in my car. I was so paranoid before. I used to wear a gun when I went out to get the mail."

Over the next few years he did well, requiring a single dose of *Mercurius sulphuricum* infrequently. At one point he was so well I did not see him for six years as his allergies were mild to non-existent.

In 2006, he told me he had given up his handgun in 2003. Though his suspicious nature was far less he did admit, "When I go in a restaurant, I scan the place to look for anyone who could be a threat."

It is hard to know whether scanning a restaurant for danger is sensible or overly suspicious. I decided his suspiciousness was more than average and *Mercurius sulphuricum* was repeated.

A year and a half later, in June, 2008, I saw him again. He said his allergies were now extremely mild. "I can't tell you the last time I was sick," he said. Since I last saw him, I had written up his case history and let him read it. He looked astonished as he read. "It's amazing how I've changed," he said. "I've come a long way." I agreed.

In October, 2011, he came in for an unrelated matter, hydrocele of the testes. We spoke of how he was fourteen years ago. "In retrospect," he said, "that was quite shocking—that I had that kind of paranoia. It makes me wonder if it was really me."

"Do you still keep a firearm?" I asked.

"I have a gun I keep in the house for protection," he said, "but I can't remember the last time I looked at it."

So, yes, paranoia and allergies can be related. And, they can be cured **at the same time and with the same** medicine. Homeopathy is a therapeutic science designed to skillfully treat the person first, the illness second. Put the person right and the illnesses will come right, too.

twenty six

Two Separate Disorders, Each Severe, Both Better with One Medicine

When a patient has more than one disorder and each is severe, the correctly prescribed homeopathic medicine will eliminate them both. Yes, both disorders will go away. And no, I am not exaggerating.

To explain how two very different diseases can be removed in one fell swoop, i.e., one homeopathic medicine, we have to revisit two of Hahnemann's concepts, the **Totality of the symptoms** and the **Vital Force**. Remember, the Vital Force is one seamless energy field surrounding and penetrating the physical body. In health, it is in dynamic order (*dynamis* = *subtle force*). In illness, it is in dynamic disorder. When disordered, it produces symptoms that are not necessarily confined to one of the body's systems (respiratory, nervous, endocrine, musculoskeletal, etc.) Often, many areas are affected. The homeopathic medicine treats the disordered Vital Force, restoring it to order and it, in turn, affects the physical, material body turning it into order. Order is health. To do this we rely on as many symptoms as we can get, particularly those that are a bit strange. All those symptoms, taken together, we refer to as the **totality of the symptoms**. When the vital energy is in order, morbid disorders (diseases) subside and disappear. In the case that follows, one homeopathic medicine cured both epilepsy and asthma.

Epilepsy, for centuries, has been a dreaded disease. Its hallmark is that it strikes without warning rendering the victim temporarily helpless. Epilepsy is a generic term used to define a family of seizure disorders. A seizure is a disturbance of the electrical activity of the brain. Usually it is brief. A person with recurrent seizures is said to have epilepsy. In all seizures, from very mild to the extreme 'grand mal' type all the customary control that the cerebral cortex normally exerts is suddenly suspended. Bundles of neurons fire uncontrollably causing lack of awareness and involuntary movements. These out of control movements convulse the victim causing him to shake, tremble or spasm sometimes slowly, usually rapidly and violently.

Bella, age two years nine months, was brought in by her grandmother, Mildred, in January, 2008. Mildred said the seizures began when was she was three weeks of age. The first two were of the grand mal type with opisthotonous and loss of consciousness. Opisthotonous is when the convulsion causes a violent spasm arching the back. At the same time the arms extend violently, the wrists flex, and the heels flex toward the back. She was prescribed phenobarbital which did not stop the seizures. After those first two grand mal seizures, the seizures changed: the head extended backward, the eyes rolled up and backwards, the lips protruded. "She pooches them out," were Mildred's words. Sometimes she lost consciousness. If she was standing, the head extended backwards and she often fell back unconscious. These were occurring every two to three days though yesterday she had had two and had already had one the morning I saw her.

After briefly being given phenobarbital as an infant, Mildred decided against further pharmaceuticals and Bella had never been medicated since. I asked Mildred why she was so strongly opposed to drugs. Seizures can be worrisome if not terrifying and even the anti drug crowd usually will allow one or more anti-seizure medicines.

"I won't allow it," she said. "I don't believe in drugs." Her unswerving point of view had resulted in more than one medical doctor calling Child Protective Services of the State of Texas. From the conventional doctor's point of view Mildred's actions were unreasoning, unethical and very possibly injurious to Bella's health and well-being. Mildred got investigated twice and twice prevailed. Bella was permitted to stay with her grandmother.

So Mildred brought Bella to me in a drug free state which meant that any symptoms I uncovered were a natural product of her disease. That is to say, the Vital Force, the electromagnetic field within and without the physical body, was not in a state of balance and harmony but instead was disordered producing the abnormal electrical activity in the brain which In turn was producing the seizures. When a patient is not taking pharmaceuticals, which is unusual, the symptoms produced by the illness are reliable. When a patient is taking a pharmaceutical one can never be sure if a symptom is drug induced or produced by the illness.

Back to Bella. Her seizures, when I first saw her, were as described above but in the past month there had been a change. Now they were followed by sleepiness. During a seizure, said Mildred, Bella's breathing would stop for a few seconds and her face would go either pale or gray. The lips became dark blue or purple. Also, there was blueness around the mouth.

I asked about Bella's parents. Her father, a Mexican-American, was in jail for drunk driving. Her Caucasian mother, who lived in the same house with Mildred and Bella, was so depressed that she showed little or no interest in her daughter. Mildred, by default, was Bella's real mother.

I needed more clues. I wanted to know about Bella's birth. She was born vaginally. I wanted to know was the cord around her neck? It was not. "But she was gasping for breath and she was very cold," recounted Mildred. "Almost blue." Bluish skin is due to insufficient oxygen in the blood and is known as *cyanosis.* The doctors gave her oxygen and warmed her up and placed her in intensive care for three days.

The cyanosis at birth, not a healthy sign, interested me. Could she have received too little oxygen in those first moments possibly damaging the brain, setting the stage for seizures?

I then learned Bella's fingertips and nail beds turned blue during her seizures. So the color blue signifying cyanosis was an ongoing symptom that began at birth.

Bella had another problem: asthma. It was diagnosed when she was one though before then doctors spoke vaguely of "breathing difficulties." Despite the grandmother's dislike of anti-epileptic drugs she allowed Bella to use a breathing machine with albuterol, a common inhaled medicine for asthma.

"She will start coughing and wheezing," said Mildred, "and if I don't' get her on the breathing machine right away her lips and face, especially the lips, will go blue. Also her fingertips."

Again, the blueness. Bella reacted swiftly to a decrease in oxygen by becoming cyanotic whether with asthma or with a seizure.

There was something else quite strange. Since the day she was born, she would stop breathing if she was placed on her back. Even now, when on her back, a rattling sound occurred as she breathed. This anomaly is quite inexplicable physiologically. But an anomaly is what makes homeopathic diagnosis interesting. The homeopath looks in his many books of symptoms to see if it has been observed before. A homeopath cannot claim to understand the anomaly physiologically, but he can accept it. He can wonder if during some proving somewhere another person manifested the same anomaly. If so, it could provide the crucial clue leading to the curative medicine.

I asked about her disposition and learned she was a mostly happy child and quite intelligent. She had potty trained herself early and had learned her ABC's from her older sister.

I inquired about foods and learned she craved sour pickles. She often ate three or four three-inch pickles a day. "She'd eat more if I let her," said Mildred.

Bella's symptoms were starting to make sense. In the rubric, "Respiration difficult in newborns," there are only two medicines and one of them is *Antimonium tartaricum.* In the provings, this medicine produces bluish lips, rattling respiration, sleepiness with bronchial inflammation and a strong desire for sour foods. So I had a pretty good match in *Antimonium tartaricum.* Were there possibly other symptoms that Bella had that I had no good way of inquiring about?

To see, I opened the *Materia Medica* by William Boericke, M.D. to *Antimonium tartaricum.* Boericke wrote that *Antimonium tartaricum* has "incessant quivering of the chin.

"Did you ever notice any quivering with Bella?" I asked. "Yes, before she has a seizure, her chin often quivers," said Mildred, "and sometimes before a severe asthma attack." Bingo! I had an unusual confirmatory symptom. What I had done was to inquire about a symptom that I had not observed nor had the grandmother volunteered. But a quivering chin can occur in patients who need *Antimonium tartaricum.* By reading Boericke's *Materia Medica* I was able to find that out, ask about it and confirm that she needed *Antimonium tartaricum.*

Antimonium tartaricum is also known to produce sleepiness. So I asked about that. "Well, yes," said Mildred. "She can be sitting at a table and suddenly nod off."

What about the fact she could not breathe well lying on her back? I looked up "Asthmatic respiration worse lying on the back"; "Difficult respiration lying on the back," and "Respiration rattling, worse lying on the back" and in none of those three rubrics does *Antimonium tartaricum* appear. No matter. The *totality of the symptoms* clearly pointed to *Antimonium tartaricum* and it is the totality of symptoms that Samuel Hahnemann said was all important. In the seventh paragraph of his seminal work, Organon of Medicine, Hahnemann wrote: "...the totality of the symptoms must be the principal, indeed the only, thing the physician has to take note of in every case of disease and to remove by means of his art, in order that the disease shall be cured and transformed into health."

Bella received *Antimonium tartaricum* 30c, a single dose.

A chat by telephone with Mildred six weeks later revealed that Bella had one more seizure that occurred a day after *Antimonium tartaricum* and none since. Also, two days after *Antimonium tartaricum* her asthma ceased.

"Before you treated her," said Mildred, "she was sleepy often during the day. Now she is full of life and active."

Nine months later

No seizures. No asthma. Perfectly healthy. Pickle consumption down to one a day.

What is so interesting about Bella's case is that one homeopathic medicine, *Antimonium tartaricum*, could remove such apparently divergent conditions as seizures and asthma. And do so in a dilution of 1/1,000,000,000,000,000,000,000,000,000,000. Yes, that is a fraction containing thirty zeros! Conventional or allopathic medicine can never reconcile that a seizure disorder and a respiratory disorder, in this case asthma, could possibly be related. After all, there are neurologists and pulmonologists and, apparently, never the twain shall meet.

If an event like the disappearance of seizures and asthma can occur simultaneously and it most certainly did occur in Bella, then we must rethink medicine and we must rethink the way the body functions.

To repeat myself yet again (Chapter one), it is clear there has to be a subtle energetic field within and without the perceivable body and this field strongly influences the physical body. It is the all-powerful Vital Force. It can be influenced in two major ways.

1. By all manner of illness.
2. By homeopathic medicines.

In the first instance, an illness (be it trauma, a virus, a bacteria, a fungus or a genetic disorder) disturbs the Vital Force. Once disturbed, the Vital Force produces symptoms. These symptoms can be anywhere from the mind and emotions to any part of the physical body.

In the second instance, homeopathic medicines also influence the Vital Force. When ingested by a healthy person they produce symptoms that were not present before taking the medicine. This is known as a proving.

When the Vital Force has been disturbed or disordered by an illness, the correct homeopathic medicine, i.e., that which most closely corresponds in its proving symptoms to the symptoms of the illness, will remove the disorder restoring harmony to the Vital Force. The Vital Force, now more coherent and unified, in turn causes the biochemistry and physiology to become normal and the illness to disappear.

twenty seven

Can homeopathic medicine cure problems which are strictly mechanical, for example, pain caused by a relatively hard part of the body (bone, cartilage) pressing on a softer part (nerve)? Yes, it can. Compression of the sciatic nerve can cause such a pain and the correct homeopathic medicine can remedy it as the case below shows.

SCIATICA AND ALLERGIES CURED WITH TELLURIUM

Sciatica is a common back problem with one to five people suffering from it at some point in their lives. The sciatic nerves, one on each side, come off the spinal cord in the low back and travel through the buttocks and down the lower extremities. When compressed, irritation ensues and then pain which can be severe. The pain often extends from the low back down to the feet. Numbness and tingling may or may not accompany it. Though most cases of sciatica resolve on their own within four weeks, a substantial number do not. It is thought the main cause of sciatica is a protrusion of a lower lumbar disc pressing on one or the other of the sciatic nerves. Sciatica is invariably one-sided. An uncommon cause of sciatica is stenosis or narrowing of the spinal canal. Also uncommon is when the sciatic nerve runs through the piriformis muscle rather than beneath it. It is presumed the piriformis spasms or tightens around the sciatic nerve causing pain. The most common cause of sciatica, however, is protrusion or herniation of a lumbar disk causing compression on and pain in the sciatic nerve. When the disc protrusion becomes extreme, surgery may be necessary.

Chiropractic manipulation can shorten the course of sciatica as can various physiotherapy techniques. Both approaches rely on mechanical movement to counter the compression on the sciatic nerve. Homeopathy does not. The homeopathic medicine is highly diluted and succussed (Chapter Two). Each medicine has a different energetic configuration depending on the substance from which it was derived. As mentioned before, these medicines act on the Vital Force putting it into a state of harmonious balance. Thus, the newly invigorated Vital Force acts on the physiological and biochemical substrates which in turn heal the disorder.

Marta, a sixty-five year old woman, had been suffering from right-sided sciatic pain since July, 1996. I saw her one year later, in July, 1997. The pain travelled from the low back down the back of the thigh to the ankle. She could only fall asleep on her left side and if she turned on to the right, the pain woke her. The pain was worse lifting a moderately heavy suitcase, worse sneezing and worse straining at stool. Her symptoms corresponded to *Tellurium* an element on the periodic table. In its homeopathic form, *Tellurium* is known to alleviate sciatica which is worse from coughing and straining. Curiously, it is known to act on right-sided sciatica.

Many homeopathic medicines predominantly affect either the right or the left side of the body. Skillful homeopaths pay close attention to laterality. When most of a patient's symptoms point to a certain medicine but the laterality does not correspond, then it probably should be discarded.

In July, 1997, she was given a single dose of *Tellurium* 200c and improved dramatically within days. Seven months later, she relapsed. She noted she had to sleep in a semi-reclined position, otherwise, on waking and rising from bed she experienced a sharp, sudden pain that began in the low back and extended down the right leg. As before, the pain was worse from coughing, sneezing and pressing at stool. She also mentioned she liked apples. It so happens that in the proving of *Tellurium* some provers experienced a desire to eat apples. So, once again her symptoms fit *Tellurium*, including a desire for apples. Two days after another dose, she was able to sleep flat and rise from bed without pain. At one month, she was seventy-five percent better. She went on to a full recovery. Again in 2012 she had a recurrence of the right-sided sciatic pain and again *Tellurium* put her right within days.

Tellurium is one of the lesser used homeopathic medicines and has won most of its laurels in the treatment of sciatic nerve pain. As always in homeopathy, *Tellurium* will not cure all or even most sciatic nerve pains. The homeopath must inquire into all aspects of the pain and the person.

In the case of Marta, *Tellurium* acted so swiftly and her improvement was so dramatic that when she came to me in February, 1998, for allergies and loss of voice, I thought I'd give *Tellurium* a try even though it is not well-known in that area. Again, it acted with the allergies ceasing with a few days.

The conclusion I drew from treating both Marta's right-sided sciatica and her allergies was that *Tellurium* was probably her **constitutional** medicine, that is, a medicine that corresponded so well to Marta that it acted curatively in two quite separate conditions. Virtually all doctors, excepting homeopaths, would say that sciatica and allergies are not known to be related. Homeopaths believe that all illnesses, all complaints, are connected.

When one medicine acts time and again to alleviate a medical problem, be it emotional or physical, we call that medicine his or her **constitutional** medicine.

twenty eight

Homeopathy In Life-Threatening Infections

Most of this book has dealt with chronic disease. What about life-threatening acute illnesses? Most homeopaths never get the opportunity to treat such cases as the patients inevitably end up in the hospital. If homeopathy is to be taken seriously, it must be shown to act effectively in life-threatening acute illnesses. An **acute illness** is of short duration ending in either death or recovery.

ACUTE PNEUMONIA TREATED WITH PHOSPHORUS

A fifty-one year old woman called me from the hospital. "I was hospitalized yesterday because I have pneumonia," she said. "I am on antibiotics and not getting better. Can you help?"

"Tell me what happened," I said.

She told how her illness began three days earlier with fever, chills and headache beginning around 3 p.m. and continuing all night. The next morning she awoke without symptoms but by the afternoon the same symptoms returned. On the third day, she went to a clinic. A chest x-ray showed pneumonia of the right upper lobe. Because her spleen had been removed some years before, her immune system was thought to be compromised. She was therefore hospitalized. Antibiotics were started immediately. That night she had an intense headache. "My head felt on fire," she said. "They brought me an ice pack but it didn't help."

With pneumonia, it is helpful for the homeopath to know which part of the lung is affected as there are homeopathic medicines specific for the right lung, left lung, right upper lobe, right lower lobe, etc. As her chest x-ray showed right upper lobe involvement, that would influence my choice of homeopathic medicine.

"Tell me your current symptoms," I said.

"Well, I have not been short of breath."

Most unusual. Virtually all patients with pneumonia have difficulty breathing *unless* the pneumonia is confined to one of the two upper lobes. These upper lobes usually come into play with exertion, when more oxygen is required. She was at bed rest.

"What else?"

"Well, I have a chill that runs up my back. It comes every two to three hours."

"What about your thirst?" I wanted to know.

"I am very thirsty, drinking two to three cups every hour."

"You want the water cold or room temperature?"

"I'd like it room temperature, but they bring it cold. Doesn't matter, I still drink a lot."

"Do you feel better lying in one position or the other?"

"Well, I feel better lying on my right," she said.

"Anything else?" I asked. "Do you want to be left alone or do you want visitors?"

"I'd just as soon be alone," she said.

"Why is that?"

"Well, when people are talking, it's just too noisy," she said.

To treat pneumonia, the homeopath looks to see what distinguishes one pneumonia from another. For the conventional M.D. the only thing that counts is to know if it is viral or bacterial and if the latter, which bacteria is responsible so that the correct antibiotic can be selected. For the homeopath, everything is in the details. As we mentioned earlier, we have medicines that favor different sides of the lung, that are thirsty, thirstless, that are worse lying on one side or the other and so on and so forth.

The fact her pneumonia was right-sided was a good starting point. But the most unusual symptom was the chill which started in the low back and travelled up the back occurring every two to three hours. That she felt better lying on her right side was also important.

I consulted the Repertory and found the following rubrics:

- Head pain burning, as if the brain were on fire.
- Chest - inflammation, lungs, right.
- Back - coldness, extending up the back.
- Lying on the right side ameliorates.
- Thirst, extreme with fever.
- Sensitive to noise.
- Aversion to company.

Using these rubrics, two medicines emerged: *Phosphorus* and *Sulphur*. They appeared to be of equal importance. Because people needing *Phosphorus* are known to have high thirst during fever and those needing Sulphur not, she was given *Phosphorus*.

I spoke to her the following morning, less than eighteen hours after taking *Phosphorus*.

"I think you hit it out of the ballpark," she said. "Within an hour I began to feel better. I had no fever all night. No cough."

"What about that funny chill in the back?"

"No chills at all," she said.

Her energy was good. "I'm walking around. I'm ready to go."

It is fascinating how the allopath and the homeopath approach pneumonia. Look up pneumonia on the internet and you will find these symptoms:

- Fever
- Cough
- Shortness of breath
- Sweating
- Chills
- Chest pain, often with each breath
- Headache
- Muscle pains
- Fatigue
- Chest x-ray showing radiographic evidence of the infection

Notice that all the symptoms are common to pneumonia. The homeopath has no problem with the allopathic diagnosis. In fact, he is in agreement with it.

The homeopath, however, wants to know more. He is interested in the details. In the case of my patient, it was important which side of the lungs was affected because we have medicines known to affect different parts of the lungs. The chill was striking because it moved **up** the back. A limited number of homeopathic medicines have such a chill, one of which is *Phosphorus.* Also, *Phosphorus* patients invariably feel worse lying on the left and better on the right. In addition, they are very thirsty. Usually, patients needing *Phosphorus* want company, want people nearby and want attention, even affection. She did not. A small subset of persons needing *Phosphorus* prefers to be alone. She was one of those.

Hers was a life-threatening pneumonia. However, the correct homeopathic medicine caused a rapid, dramatic improvement.

Because she was in hospital and on IV antibiotics, they were continued but the dramatic improvement after *Phosphorus* which occurred within one hour suggested that it was homeopathic *Phosphorus* that enabled her recovery to be dramatic and quick.

So, yes, even in acute pneumonia, homeopathy can be effective.

twenty nine

Homeopathy Can Be Useful even when Critical Parts of the Body have been Surgically Removed

In the following example, a woman improved significantly with homeopathic treatment when there was no plausible physiological explanation.

SHORT GUT SYNDROME
CHRONIC DIARRHEA STOPPED WITH CROTON TIGLIUM

She had no ileum, a three and a half to four meter long piece of the small intestine. It had been surgically removed over four years before. As a result, she was having frequent diarrhea and had to be extremely careful about everything she put in her mouth. She was seventy years old and I had earlier treated her successfully for the skin condition known as urticaria or hives.

The ileum is the third portion of the small intestine. Its wall is made up of many folds containing villi–minute, finger-like projections capable of absorbing large quantities of the products of digestion, namely, bile salts and vitamin B-12. It also secretes many enzymes crucial in the digestion of protein and carbohydrate. The ileum also absorbs fatty acids. Because of the villi, the ileum presents a vast surface for absorption. When the ileum is removed, the partially processed products of digestion go straight into the colon or large intestine. The result: frequent diarrhea and vitamin B-12 deficiency requiring life-long supplementation.

My patient suffered from trigger-quick diarrhea. Daily she had diarrhea immediately after eating or drinking. She had to be constantly vigilant to drink small quantities and eat small portions. Anything more set off diarrhea within minutes. She had what is known as "Short Gut Syndrome" or "Short Bowel Syndrome."

The question: could homeopathy help in spite of the fact she was missing a long, crucial segment of the small intestine? I thought it worth a try and took the following symptoms from the Repertory:

- Diarrhea immediately after eating.
- Diarrhea immediately after drinking.
- Diarrhea, sudden.

These symptoms suggested the homeopathic medicine, *Croton tiglium* which is made from croton oil. Croton oil is a powerful purgative, causing the stool to be evacuated in a sudden gush, like a shot. My patient described her diarrhea in just those terms. When croton oil is prepared homeopathically, it has the potential to reverse and cure sudden, gushing diarrhea.

She took a single dose and **the diarrhea ceased**. She was able to eat and drink normally.

This kind of result cannot be satisfactorily explained physiologically. The loss of the ileum means the loss of the existing gut's ability to absorb nutrients. Usually, after the removal of the ileum, the remaining gut partially takes over some of the duties of the ileum. This adaptation takes about two years and even then most people with no ileum still have diarrhea. Some even need parenteral (intravenous) nutrition. My patient's diarrhea went away within a few days and her operation had been four years earlier.

My explanation: *Croton tiglium*–an energetic trace of croton oil–re-ordered the vital energy or Vital Force, putting it into dynamic balance. The now revivified Vital Force then exerted its influence on the existing gut causing it to act and work normally.

The annals of homeopathy contain innumerable unlikely cures and that is what spurs homeopaths the world over never to say never and always to offer hope.

But my patient may not have needed to have her ileum removed. Here is the rest of the story.

In 2006, she was diagnosed with endometrial cancer. The uterus and both ovaries were surgically removed. She then underwent chemotherapy and radiation therapy. "It took me two years to recuperate," she said. "And then I needed supplemental potassium and a B-12 shot once a month in addition to Loperamide to control the diarrhea."

It was the radiation that nearly did her in. "As I was nearing the end of the radiation treatments in 2007, I knew I had had enough. I was sure the radiation treatments were harming me. I begged my doctors not to do anymore."

She was part of a research protocol which called for chemotherapy and radiation therapy in addition to surgery. As she was one of only five patients with the exact same pathology, the doctors were adamant she continue and refused her request.

"I told them, 'I'm not coming back.' Then they said they'd bring the radiation equipment to my house. My answer: 'I'll tell the people at the gate not to let you in.' Then they shifted from trying to persuade me to persuading my husband. They told him, 'If she doesn't receive the radiation the cancer will return and we won't be able to stop it.'

"So I consented. I lay on the table crying. About three months later, if I swallowed food, I'd vomit it up so violently it would end up across the room. I went back to the hospital for a barium swallow. I couldn't keep the barium down. Then they did a CT scan which showed the ileum was non-functioning. Four days later, I was in surgery and they removed the ileum."

That is how she ended up with Short Gut Syndrome and daily diarrhea, extra potassium daily and a monthly shot of B-12. Could things have worked out differently? It's hard to know. The doctors were wedded to their research protocol and refused to alter it. Yet she knew the radiation was harming her. Why is it is difficult for doctors to listen to patients? Hers is not an isolated incidence. Legions of patients tell me similar stories–that their doctors don't listen and, when they do, discount what they have to say.

Had she not had the final radiation treatments, would the cancer have returned? No one will ever know. The surgeon cleaned up the mess caused by too much radiation and, incredibly, homeopathic *Croton tiglium* was able to undo some of the havoc caused by the loss of her ileum.

thirty

It can be difficult to distinguish a patient who says he is depressed from one who is simply exhausted. Even seasoned medical doctors and psychologists can be misled. Often, with homeopathic treatment, as the person's energy improves, their "apparent" depression vanishes. It can be a tough call as the following case report illustrates.

DEPRESSED OR EXHAUSTED? A CASE OF GELSEMIUM

"I don't know what's wrong with Dov," she said on the phone. "I think he's depressed. He's definitely not himself. He's not getting up until one in the afternoon, sometimes, two or three. Or he gets up and goes back to bed. He has no interest in anything. He just mopes around the house."

I had known Dov for over nine years. He was one of the most energetic men I knew. In fact, he could be downright boisterous with his enthusiasm and joie de vivre.

I called Dov. "I'm tired all the time," he said. "I get up at 2 p.m. My eyes want to close. If I get out of bed at 8:30 or 9:00 I want to go back to bed. My eyelids are heavy."

Dov was an avid motorcycle rider. He loved riding for miles in the open air.

I asked him if he was riding. "No. I'm exhausted. The very idea of suiting up and wheeling it out is exhausting."

I asked if he was getting out and seeing people. "I don't make any effort to be around people," he said. "I avoid people and I feel lonely."

He only felt happy around his wife, whom he adored. "When I found Joline, I found my soul mate. She is my world. I stay with her until I fall asleep."

He continued on about his physical state. "I feel weak in general. If I have to stoop down to look for something under the bed, it's an effort. I am not fluid. It is a series of movements. Each act is hard. I have to tell my body what to do. It used to be fluid. Now it is not. My body feels weak. I walk slowly. I'm not walking well. I'm less fluid."

Joline added, "When he walks he doesn't lift up his legs like he used to. His posture is slumped."

Dov then said, "I know underneath this layer, I am sane." My mind is good."

So there it was. He was stating clearly that he was not depressed, simply exhausted. His use of the word "fluid" was peculiar. He used it several times saying his body did not feel "fluid," nor were his movements "fluid." I thought of the rubric in the Repertory, "Will, muscles refuse to obey the will when attention is turned away." Though he did not use those words, he conveyed that idea when he said, "I have to tell my body what to do."

The principal medicine for this peculiar state is *Gelsemium sempervirens. Gelsemium*, also known as Yellow Jasmine, is known for producing and curing exhaustion so extreme that even the simplest of movements require unusual attention. It is also useful when the body feels extremely heavy, especially the eyelids.

I sent Dov *Gelsemium*, a single dose.

We spoke two weeks later. "I am one hundred per cent better," he said. "After I took your medicine, I got a severe headache and could not sleep. Within two days my energy returned. I am getting up in the morning, full of energy. Now I realize how bad I was. I was tired all the time. Now I feel great. Today, I got up at 6 a.m. and started cleaning the kitchen. I want to do things. My wife said, 'Dr. Robinson overdid it!' It's a huge change. I'm very thankful."

Gelsemium is, perhaps, our leading medicine for influenza as it corresponds to the extreme weakness and exhaustion produced by influenza. Many patients with the flu who need *Gelsemium* will say how heavy the body feels, how hard it is to keep the eyelids open. Sometimes, the weakness can be so advanced that the legs will tremble on getting out of a chair or even walking.

The fact that Dov had a headache just after taking *Gelsemium* suggested that the medicine was causing an **aggravation** meaning that the patient gets worse in some way before getting better. It is a sign the medicine is working and one can expect a favorable outcome.

Remember, these homeopathic medicines produce symptoms in healthy persons and then cure those same symptoms when they appear in illness (Like cures like).

thirty one

The human body is so incredibly complex that discoveries concerning how it functions in health and disease will continue, perhaps forever. The following case report has to do with muscle wasting, but, unexpected, only the upper body lost flesh. Currently, there is no scientific explanation for this phenomenon though, interestingly, homeopaths over one hundred years ago observed and treated it.

MUSCLE WASTING (SARCOPENIA) AND WEAKNESS OF THE UPPER BODY DISAPPEARING WITH SALT

It was strange—his change in health. Over the past several months, he had noticed a drastic loss in his physical strength, **but only in the upper body.** I had known this seventy-seven-year-old man for years. He had always been robust and, until a few years ago, had competed in Team Penning, a physically demanding rodeo sport demanding stamina, coordination and team work.

In team penning, three mounted riders have to pick three numbered cattle out of a herd of thirty, cut the three loose from the other twenty-seven, and herd them as fast as possible into a pen at the other end of the arena, all the while making sure none of the other twenty-seven cross a foul line. If the team takes more than ninety seconds, it is automatically disqualified. Team penning requires horse and rider to break into an instant gallop, stop abruptly, and wheel the horse in a tight turn.

As my patient recounted it: "You're whippin' and ridin,' stoppin' and startin.' These horses are wide-open galloping and then stoppin' and turning on a dime. The hardest part is staying in the saddle. Every second counts."

In 1997, his team, which included his wife, won the National Team Pin Championship. He continued to compete until he was seventy-two.

After that he continued to do very hard outdoor, physical work. His loss of strength was most unexpected.

"Lately, I have been waking at 3:30 a.m. from muscle pain," he said. "My energy level collapses during the day. It drops suddenly—within minutes—and I have to go home and nap. My upper body is turning to flab. My strength is way down. It is hard for me to lift twenty-five pounds.

The strange part was that the **weakness was confined to the upper body with the lower limbs as strong as ever**. He was sensitive to the heat and avoided it. He would get a headache within one minute of exposure to the summer sun. He also mentioned some painful blisters in the right side of the scalp.

Muscle wasting is associated with aging and medical science can do little more than describe it. It is sometimes called **sarcopenia**, defined as loss of skeletal muscle mass and strength associated with aging. Lack of exercise is thought to be a significant factor in the development of sarcopenia. My patient, however, had continued to exercise faithfully all the while losing muscle mass and strength.

There are two homeopathic medicines known for loss of strength and wasting of the muscles in the upper body with the lower limbs remaining strong and healthy. They are *Lycopodium* (prepared from Club Moss) and *Natrum muriaticum,* (a homeopathic preparation of **salt**). Lycopodium usually craves sugar and sweets, *Natrum muriaticum* craves salt.

He was not much interested in sweets. "What about salt?" I asked.

"I don't eat it. When I do, I swell up immediately—my feet and fingers. For fifty years I have avoided salt."

People needing *Natrum muriaticum* often crave salt and use a lot of it. A subset cannot tolerate salt. He fit into the latter category. These people usually are hot and dislike the heat. Exposure to the sun often brings on a headache. He fit all the criteria.

He was given a single dose of *Natrum muriaticum* in September, 2011. We spoke a month later. "I think my body structure is changing—it is correcting itself," he said. "The tissue under the abdomen was loose and sagging. Now it is not sagging as much. And I can lift more than I could. I feel stronger."

He spoke of his arms. "Before this medicine," he said "they were wrinkled and flabby and hanging down like a little old lady. Now they are beginning to firm up. Before, I was doing a fifteen minute workout on an exercise machine but it didn't matter. The arms got more and more flabby and weak."

His wife told how his color had improved. "Before this treatment," she said, "he looked terrible. You know, Dr. Robinson, I think his upper body weakness actually began in the fall of 2009."

"I am definitely stronger than I was," he said, "unless I eat bread. Another thing. I still need to take a nap but now I notice it's when I've eaten bread." So, he was sensitive to wheat. This was not surprising. Many people are sensitive to wheat. Especially those people needing *Natrum muriaticum.* Because he was starting to improve, I knew *Natrum muriaticum* was the correct medicine. It would be a matter of time until he regained full strength and muscle mass and, perhaps, even the ability to tolerate wheat. The painful blisters in the scalp disappeared four days after *Natrum muriaticum.*

When we spoke again a month later, he was sleeping better. "I can now lift fifty pounds," he said. There was no more muscle pain. He still could not tolerate wheat.

Over the next few months, he noted he was standing straighter. His energy continued to improve. "I used to come home and go to sleep immediately. Now, I come home and do things—work the horses, cut down trees. My chest is back up where it should be and my abdomen is hanging down less. I can lift fifty pounds many times in a day now."

His urination was improving. "Used to be I'd get the urge to urinate but the stream was weak. Now, when I get up at 5 a.m. I'm able to pee better."

Such is the wonder of homeopathy. Not only was his muscle strength improving but also his energy, sleep, muscle pain, posture, ability to walk and to urinate. And all these improvements from a homeopathic dilution of salt! And how ironic it is that people needing

Natrum muriaticum often love salt and eat a lot of it. Or, like my patient, they do not tolerate it.

Why these people lose flesh beginning in the neck and moving down cannot be explained by modern physiology but it was observed over two hundred years ago by homeopaths.

Had my patient not been treated with *Natrum muriaticum* his muscle wasting and weakness would have certainly progressed, debilitating him further and further. He received *Natrum muriaticum* once a month for several months and then, as he was so much better, it was stopped.

Homeopathy—it cures even where modern medicine has no clear understanding of the pathophysiology and no cure.

An interesting footnote: In 2001, he complained of recurrent severe muscle cramps which would begin with the fingers and toes curling, followed by a fierce spasm beginning in the legs that would move up the inner thighs to the groin and up the trunk pulling his head and chest down onto his thighs. "It felt like the tendons were being pulled out with pliers," he recounted. "I couldn't straighten up, let alone walk. I would scream in pain." Ironically, if he ate a little salt or salt and baking soda (sodium bicarbonate), the spasms went off in a few minutes. In that situation, salt was needed and cured without causing swelling. At all other times his system did not tolerate salt. Salt, sodium chloride, is indispensable to all living cells and virtually all foods contain salt. My patient was and is exquisitely sensitive to too little or too much salt.

thirty two

Vertigo, with the world spinning around you, is intensely uncomfortable. It is not easy to control it with conventional medicine.

The person will report that either the world seems to be spinning or he, himself, is spinning. A spinning sensation, therefore, is common to vertigo. It is difficult to prescribe on common symptoms as there are over six hundred homeopathic medicines that can treat vertigo. The trick, then, is to find one homeopathic medicine that closely corresponds to the person suffering from vertigo. To do so requires careful questioning of the patient and a detailed knowledge of the various homeopathic medicines.

True vertigo is not the same as dizziness which is a feeling of lightheadedness or a faint feeling. Dizziness can occur from an emotional upset such as the sight of blood, from standing up too quickly, or from an illness such as the flu. Vertigo is significantly worse than dizziness and people with vertigo cannot walk or drive. It is sometimes referred to as "Benign Paroxysmal Positional Vertigo."

The homeopath does not treat vertigo per se, but instead pays attention to the symptoms accompanying the vertigo. As the accompanying symptoms will vary from one case of vertigo to the next, so will the curative homeopathic medicine vary.

A CASE OF THE SPINNING ILLNESS

A fifty-two-year-old woman caught cold and within three days developed debilitating vertigo. She had nausea with the vertigo. The vertigo was worse looking at something moving. Nausea with vertigo is common, vertigo worse when looking at a moving object is more unusual. As the mental state is often the key to a successful prescription, I asked about stress. It turned out her daughter had given birth to a baby girl, her first granddaughter, a month earlier. Her daughter was behaving irresponsibly, going out at night with her girlfriends to drink beer and coming in late. Other evenings, she took the small baby with her when she left to hang out with her friends. My patient was worried more for her granddaughter than her daughter. One night, her daughter came in after 1 a.m., and she only got three and a half hours of sleep. Two days later the vertigo began.

Her loss of sleep leading to vertigo was an important symptom. So was her worry and anxiety for her tiny granddaughter. These two factors pointed to *Cocculus indicus*. *Cocculus* also has vertigo worse from looking at a moving object.

She mentioned she had a lifelong tendency to carsickness and *Cocculus* is one of the principle medicines for motion sickness.

I consulted the Repertory and used the following rubrics:

- Vertigo after loss of sleep.
- Vertigo looking at a moving object.
- Vertigo and nausea from riding in a car.

All rubrics contained *Cocculus* which was given.

Twelve hours later, she reported the vertigo was mostly gone. "It's better, a lot better," she said, "though I still have to be careful not to move too quickly." Her head continued to feel "heavy," a symptom she had not mentioned the day before but which is part of *Cocculus* symptomatology. Her appetite, which had been nil, was back, strongly, always a good sign. The vertigo stayed gone and the cold slowly resolved.

A DIFFERENT VERTIGO COMBINED WITH LARYNGOSPASM

A very different vertigo required a different homeopathic medicine. A 59-year-old woman called me early one morning as I was about to board a flight to Honduras. Though I had known her for over twenty years I could barely recognize her voice which sounded as though she was being strangled. She had woken at 5 a.m. with the room spinning. She got up, took a dose of Meclizine, an antihistamine used to treat nausea, vomiting and dizziness caused by motion sickness. She went back to sleep only to wake forty-five minutes later from vertigo. "I felt the bed was spinning," she said. She was unable to stand or lie down. She vomited which immediately triggered violent spasms in the throat interfering with her speech and breathing.

As I listened to her talking, I could tell she was having trouble speaking. There was a kind of crowing sound as she breathed in. "When I inhale, I am straining to breathe," she said. "It is as if someone is squeezing my throat." The only position she could bear was sitting on the floor leaning against the bed. The vertigo was worse when she closed her eyes.

She was in a bad way suffering from what is known as "laryngospasm," where the vocal cords involuntarily contract and spasm, partially blocking the flow of air into the lungs. Laryngospasm can be caused by acid reflux. In her case, the vomitus irritated the vocal cords resulting in spasm. Laryngospasm typically subsides in a couple of minutes but her case was not typical as it was persisting.

I needed a homeopathic medicine that took into account both the vertigo and the laryngospasm. It had to act fast. Here was a situation where laryngospasm was **concomitant** to the vertigo. A concomitant symptom, in homeopathy, is one that accompanies the principal complaint, and is difficult or impossible to account for physiologically. A concomitant, therefore, is unusual and should always be taken into account when prescribing.

I consulted the repertory and chose the following rubrics (symptoms):

- Vertigo – as if everything were turning in a circle.
- Vertigo – closing the eyes aggravates.
- Throat – spasms.

The medicine selected was *Belladonna* which addressed all the symptoms. *Belladonna* is known for conditions which come on **suddenly** and violently. She took a dose (she had homeopathic medicines at home) at 7:30 a.m. Ten minutes later, she was already much better. By 10:30 a.m. she went to work.

Homeopathy: there is nothing like it in acute illness.

thirty three

Sometimes, the homeopath does not find the correct homeopathic medicine. He tries, again and again, with partial results. Then, one day, the patient mentions a salient fact and the homeopath knows precisely what medicine is needed.

THE CHILD WHO NEARLY KILLED HIS COUSIN

His name was Kurt and not only was he a patient, but a close friend whom I had been treating for the previous three years. He had had a heart attack several years before I met him and had recovered nicely after a stent was placed. He had asthma and various joint pains in the back, hips and lower extremities. He had received a number of homeopathic medicines and claimed that each one had helped him, some significantly.

One day in late 2010, he began to complain of a severe pain in the left wrist accompanied by swelling of the condyles (protuberances) of the wrist. It was a new symptom and suggested to me that he was not improving. In fact, I believed that my medicines, to date, had not been helping him. I knew I had to try again and find a homeopathic medicine that more precisely covered his symptoms. We began again to talk and he told me the following story:

"When I was five years old my parents decided to send me to live with my uncle and aunt and their two sons. At that time we were living in Tucson, Arizona. My aunt and uncle were living in Virginia, more than 2,000 miles to the east. Without telling me a thing, I was put on a train with a young woman who was my chaperone. I had no idea where we were headed but it was a great trip and I enjoyed myself immensely. One day, we arrived at this house. The woman who was taking care of me rang the bell and my aunt opened the door. My traveling companion bid me good-bye and vanished. It was quite a shock. But it got worse, much worse. My Uncle Luke had a distant manner and never showed me anything but indifference. He never treated me with affection. My oldest cousin, he was seven years older than I was, was neither friendly nor affectionate. My Aunt Ruth did little more than find jobs for me to do and issue orders. The other cousin, Billy, was 2 ½ years older than me and he really disliked me and did everything he could to make my life miserable. I remember his first words to me, 'If you touch my things, I'll kill you.' It went downhill from there.

"The atmosphere in that house was very hostile for me. Aunt Ruth was like a drill sergeant. She assigned tasks, and little else. Tessie, the German immigrant maid, played the motherly role. She was the only one who ever touched me and showed me love.

"It was in those years that I developed asthma and food allergies and became a bed wetter.

"There was one area of my life that I guarded and did not permit any meanness about. That was my mother. She was, in my mind, a sweet, distant woman. The only thing I had that was mine was my memory of my mother. It was an important, even sacred, memory for me.

"One morning, I think I was about six at the time, we were sitting at breakfast. There was Tessie, who was cooking, and Billy and me. As usual, he was giving me a hard time. He said something mean about my mother. He never said anything that was not mean.

"When he said, 'Your mother is stupid, just like you,' I said to him, 'Don't talk about my mother.'

"Tessie must have heard something in my voice. She was frying eggs. Billy acted pleased he'd found something that upset me. He kept on about my mother.

"I warned him again. 'I mean it. Lay off about my mother.' I felt tears and anger welling up. It was the one thing that belonged only to me in that house. Her specialness.

"Again, Billy persisted. He disregarded my warning and started in on my mother again.

"On the table was a steak knife. I grabbed it and lunged at his throat. The tip of the knife went into his throat about half an inch at which point Tessie's powerful hand grabbed my wrist and pulled me out of the chair. She was strong, a two hundred pound German woman. And she screamed.

"At that point, Billy began to scream and cry. He put his hand to his throat and there was a small amount of blood on his fingers.

"Tessie's screaming and Billy's screaming brought Aunt Ruth into the room. Tessie was still holding me. I'm still holding the knife. Aunt Ruth arrives and she starts screaming and rushes to her son, Billy.

"They don't know what to do with me. I'm not stopping. I'm still trying to get at him. So they decide to lock me in the pantry. They called Uncle Luke.

"I spent about two hours locked in the pantry. I remember it well. I found a fruit cake and I ate the whole thing in those two hours before they let me out. It was delicious."

Kurt had just given me a perfect description of the way a person who needs the homeopathic medicine, *Mercurius solulibis,* behaves. In fact, in the Repertory we find the following rubric: "Anger, so angry that he could have stabbed someone." *Mercurius* is there.

From that day on, Billy was careful never to push Kurt too far.

People who need *Mercurius* tend to have violent anger. They can be so angry they can punch holes in walls and their anger can translate into murderous violence.

After receiving *Mercurius,* my friend's wrist pain diminished and was gone within four to six weeks. He continued to improve. The bony swelling of the wrist went away entirely over the next six months.

It is interesting that Kurt went on to become a man unusually interested in weaponry. He has always had rifles and pistols in his house and a couple of years ago he passed an examination allowing him to carry a concealed weapon. He became an excellent shot and still is. What he learned that morning at the breakfast table as a child changed his life. At some deep level, he decided that no one, EVER, would mess with him again. "I have no intention of killing anyone. On the other hand, I will not be anyone's goddamned victim."

A single event in childhood that is drenched in strong emotion can alter one's life and, later on, lead the homeopath to a powerfully effective medicine.

thirty four

ADHD Coupled with Violent Behavior Significantly Improved with A Spider Medicine

Hyperactive children can be awfully difficult to live with and next to impossible to educate. Add in violent behavior and they can be impossible to live with.

Ana, age four, was such a child. She was brought in by her grandmother who said her granddaughter was unable to focus on anything, not even television or movies. Now, the run-of-the-mill hyperactive children with poor attention routinely cannot or will not focus on what their teachers and parents would like but invariably they possess an uncanny ability to lose themselves in one-pointed attention in television, movies and PlayStation type computer games. Not this child.

Her grandmother said she was unusually violent and would tear up books and anything else that took her fancy such as papers and virtually anything that she could tear or otherwise destroy.

"She'll take scissors and cut off her two year old sister's hair," she said. "But that's not all. She has cut the cords to TV sets, DVD players, even the xBox. Almost all the shoestrings in the house she has cut apart." She might have been destructive but she was not stupid.

She was also constantly running about in a wild fashion. As she ran about the house she would violently push chairs and tables sometimes knocking them over.

The child loved music and loved to dance. She could dance for hours. "How important is music for her? I wanted to know.

"She will seek out music," the grandmother said. "She insists on going to sleep to music."

Sleep, or the lack thereof, can provide important clues to the state of the patient and help to decide the correct homeopathic medicine.

I was interested to know if any of this whirlwind, frenetic activity persisted into sleep. "Her sleep is wild," said her grandmother. "She's more than restless. I would say she throws herself about the bed. The covers are a total mess by morning. I've noticed too that as she is falling asleep her body often jerks. It can continue while she sleeps."

Ana had a huge temper, too. "She'll kick, hit, slap and scream," said her grandmother. "She often says, 'I hate you! I hate you! Leave me alone!'" When angry her physical strength increased enormously.

She enjoyed smashing things to bits. She wrote on walls and then would break her crayons. She had broken most of her toys. She threw sticks and stones at dogs.

In perpetual fast motion, she was never still. "She's always busy," said her grandmother.

She had another peculiar quality. She was cunning. "She's very sneaky," said her grandmother. "She sneaks candy or anything else she wants. We have to keep a lock on the refrigerator." She was clever enough to get what she wanted even when her grandmother didn't want her to have it.

Her mother was severely ADD (attention deficit disorder) and was dysfunctional to the point that she allowed the grandmother full rein with her child. According to the grandmother, her daughter, the child's mother, was incapable of looking after herself much less her own children. So it was the grandmother who brought the child to me and reported the history.

In homeopathy it is always advisable to find out as many aspects of the patient as possible, not just those negative ones that brought them in the first place. "Does she have any positive qualities," I wanted to know.

"Well, yes. She likes to wash dishes and does her best at it. She also likes to fold clothes and to vacuum the floor."

After a pause, the grandmother said, "One other thing that's curious. Even when she is quite well she'll often say, 'I need to go to the doctor.'"

Indeed, that was curious. If an adult did that it would be considered a sign of hypochondriasis if not neurosis. But can a physically healthy four- year-old be neurotic? Perhaps.

But as the old refrain goes, 'Ours is not to reason why…' so the homeopath does not speculate too long on the 'why' of illness but rather stays with the concrete, the indisputable, i.e., the symptoms themselves.

We knew the child was cunning. She might have thought it cute or simply interesting to ask to go to the doctor. No matter, it was a form of feigning illness. I decided to use it as a symptom.

I needed a medicine that was wildly active, violently angry, and extremely destructive.

Looking into the Repertory the following medicines appeared: *Apis mellifica, Belladonna, Hyoscyamus, Nux-vomica, Stramonium, Sulphur, Tarentula hispanica,* and *Veratrum album.*

Finding these medicines was a good first step. Now, the problem was how to eliminate those medicines that couldn't possibly help. As always, the homeopath looks to a distinguishing feature. This child was sneaky so I decided to search for that.

The word "sneaky" is not in the Repertory but "cunning" is. There are fifteen medicines under that rubric. Even after including cunning the previous eight medicines remained active candidates.

What else could be done to winnow out the one, most similar medicine? The strong desire for music had to be taken into account. With that symptom suddenly *Tarentula hispanica,* a poisonous spider, was in first place.

But there was more. This child asked to go to the doctor. And there was nothing physically wrong with her. I looked up "Feigning illness" and there was *Tarenula hispanica.*

I again searched the Repertory and under "Destructiveness, cunning," was a single entry: *Tarentula hispanica.* This homeopathic medicine, made by serially diluting the venom of this poisonous spider, is described in Homoeopathic *Materia Medica* by William Boericke, M.D., in part as follows:

- Extreme restlessness; must keep in constant motion…
- Sudden alternation of mood.

- Foxy.
- Destructive impulses;
- Moral relaxation.
- Must constantly busy herself or walk.
- Sensitive to Music.
- Ungrateful,
- Discontented.
- Guided by whims.
- Better from music.

It seemed the perfect fit. But what about, "Sudden alternation of mood"? And then, I got it. When she wasn't running wildly, throwing fits and breaking things, she could wash dishes, fold clothes and use the vacuum—quite a turnaround from the wild, destructive side.

She received *Tarentula hispanica,* a single dose.

Seven weeks later I received the following report: "She has stopped growling," said her grandmother, much to my surprise as I was unaware of that peculiar symptom. She was no longer having temper tantrums but still could not focus when being read a story or watching a movie. She was still tearing up books, but no longer scribbling on them and she was not tearing up papers. Within the first two weeks she stopped cutting various things with scissors. She still loved music and dancing.

For two weeks she stopped running about wildly. Then the running began again. She was no longer slapping people and not flailing her arms as she had been.

"She still screams," said her grandmother, "but not nearly as often. She's no longer writing on walls but still breaking crayons." She had broken no more toys.

She was still throwing sticks and stones at dogs and kicking at them. Still very busy. Still jerking on falling asleep and during sleep. She still asked to go to the doctor when not ill.

One day her grandmother heard her say to her little sister, "Somebody needs to shoot you." She continued to tell various family members, "I hate you."

There was a new symptom: she was putting all sorts of indigestible things into her mouth and chewing on them. In the Repertory is the rubric: "Desires indigestible things" and there we find *Tarentula.*

As this particular symptom was not there before it could have been a proving symptom.

Though greatly improved, I decided to give her a second dose of *Tarentula hispanica* not only because she had a way to go but because the running wildly about had resumed after an initial improvement.

There were no further reports from her grandmother but nine months later her little sister came in for treatment for seizures and she came along.

She had been perfectly fine for months. Her former behavior had ceased entirely. No anger. No meanness. No chewing on things. No longer sneaky. Not running about wildly and no destructive behavior. "Her concentration is a hundred percent now," said her grandmother.

And all this with only two doses of *Tarentula hispanica* and there had been no other intervention either chemical (pharmacological agents) or psychotherapeutic.

Usually children with these sorts of extreme behavioral problems are treated either with a pharmacological agent to calm them down, psychotherapy with an aim to behavior modification, or a strict diet that excludes food dyes, sugary foods and any food they might be allergic to. All such treatments can be effective but none can cause such profound changes as we witnessed with the correct homeopathic medicine.

In the experience of most homeopaths, it is unusual to have such a complete, drastic turnaround with only two doses of medicine but such results buttress the idea that the **simillimum** can have utterly transformative power.

Please note: I paid little attention to the conventional diagnosis of ADHD (Attention Deficit Hyperactivity Disorder). Instead, I focused exclusively on the child's unusual symptoms. Those symptoms led to the curative medicine. It has now been over one and a half years since the girl was treated and she remains well.

thirty five

A Recurring Kidney Infection Cured with Bryonia

She came in for chronic, recurring left flank pain. Flank pain refers to pain in one side of the body between the upper abdomen and the back. It is generally a sign of kidney infection and so it was with Maria who had her first kidney infection when she was four years old. She was now nearly 31. Hospitalized in April, 2001, with chills, fever and perspiration, she was diagnosed with a kidney infection and placed on intravenous antibiotics for three days.

In September, 2002, a similar pain appeared again in the left flank and, unfortunately, it was continuing to appear, disappear and reappear. She related how the pain would come for four or five days and then disappear for eight to twelve days.

We like to think, and doctors would have us believe, that when we have an infection, we take the prescribed antibiotic and that's that. Often that is the end of it but not always. Sometimes the infection goes underground and smolders. The question is: what to do about it? Your doctor will prescribe another antibiotic, and then another, and another. This is the stage where patients become desperate and look for alternatives.

In homeopathy we approach the problem a bit differently. We have four criteria we often apply:

1. The **location** of the pain and whether or not it extends in some direction.

2. The **sensation** of the pain.
3. The **modalities** of the pain–a modality is anything that makes a symptom better or worse.
4. The **concomitants**. A concomitant is another, somewhat unusual condition that accompanies the main problem.

Her pain was located in the left flank and extended to the left upper abdomen.

The sensation she described was “pressing inwards.”

The principal modality was that it was **worse from any movement** such as walking, turning in bed, etc., and it was better lying on the painful side.

The concomitants were:

- Her urine became quite dark with each episode.
- Her thirst in the past year had increased dramatically to three liters a day—two liters of water and one of juice.
- She was perspiring more since 2001 and the sweat was oily.
- With an episode she experienced more body heat though there was no fever. Curiously, the body heat came on at bedtime around 10 p.m. and lasted until 1 a.m.

At this point I had quite an array of symptoms none of which were relevant in conventional medicine but were of key importance in my analysis.

The fact her pain was much worse from movement was important. Because it was better lying on the painful side I knew that the weight of her body on the left flank immobilized the area making movement less possible—another way of saying “worse from movement.”

Her striking increase in thirst with each episode meant that I would search for a medicine known to have increased thirst. Also, I would take into account the darker than usual urine though that was of lesser importance as it is common in kidney infections. The fact her perspiration increased and turned **oily** fascinated me. I would try to take that into account also.

So one can see that the kidney infection was having a number of different effects throughout the body—all of which were of little or no importance to the conventional doctor yet of crucial importance to the homeopath.

There had been some stress a few years back when she and her husband, both dentists, lived in Colombia before moving to the U.S. They worked with her in-laws, also dentists. The in-laws were killed in a motor vehicle accident and, as a result, they became swamped with work. Shortly afterward they began to receive a specific threat to kidnap their daughter. That proved too much and they left Colombia and moved to Florida. Suddenly, after years of hard work, there was zero work as she had no license in Florida. Her new life, without work, was very hard for her. She exercised three hours a day and worried about "not being useful."

She described herself as "hyperactive," "very strict about my values," "good manners are very important," and "responsible."

It was quite possible the stress of receiving a kidnapping threat in Colombia was setting the stage for the later breakdown of her health but there was no way to be sure of that.

I selected *Bryonia*—a medicine that covered most aspects of her illness. A *Bryonia* patient is well-known for being much, much **worse from any movement**, for having a very high thirst, dark urine and increased perspiration. I was delighted to read in the original proving of *Bryonia* by Hahnemann that it produced, "Perspiration that looked like oil..."

Very soon after taking *Bryonia* all her symptoms subsided. At a follow-up she mentioned that she felt "less over-responsible and less pressured," which suggested that *Bryonia* helped her emotionally as well as physically.

Details, minute details, such as oily perspiration only during an infection and an extreme thirst, are the building blocks of every successful homeopathic prescription. Such details are not taken into account by allopathic doctors as they consider them irrelevant. For them, there is only an infection, located in the kidney, susceptible to a certain antibiotic—end of story. When the infection keeps recurring, requiring yet another and another antibiotic, they have nothing to offer—except still another round of antibiotics.

Homeopathic medicine, carefully applied, can stimulate the body to cure itself. This is not to say every homeopathic prescription is curative. It is not. But because remarkable improvements do occur with homeopathy, it offers hope, often when conventional medicine cannot.

thirty six

Healing Fractures that Won't Heal with Homeopathy

Though this book has dealt primarily with homeopathy in the treatment of chronic disease, it can be very effective in non-chronic situations as this case report attests.

Usually fractures of the bone heal; sometimes they do not. It is when they do not that homeopathy can often help.

In June, 2008, a 60-year-old woman whom I had treated over the years called saying she had suffered a fracture of the right tibia (shin bone) after falling and landing on the right knee. An MRI (magnetic resonance imaging) confirmed the fracture.

She was having sharp pains in the right knee that were shooting back and forth. They were worse when she lay down. Also, the knee felt very hot and there was pulsating pain.

After researching the homeopathic literature, I found that *Belladonna* patients can have sharp, back and forth, transverse pains that are worse lying down. *Belladonna* is well-known for causing heat and throbbing in the affected part.

She started taking *Belladonna* as needed. After a week, the pain was much less and she could bend and extend the leg much further. By the end of July the knee pain had gone but the fracture, as determined by the x-ray taken by her orthopedic doctor, was not healing. She was very upset as he was recommending surgery.

I retook her case and decided that homeopathic calcium, known as *Calcarea carbonica*, matched her symptoms. She was given a single, highly diluted dose. In mid-August, the surgeon said the fracture was healing and by mid-October it had healed completely. Surgery avoided. Though the *Belladonna* had removed the pain, it had not touched the stubborn fracture. Only *Calcarea carbonica* was able to enable the fracture to knit together.

Calcarea carbonica will not heal all fractures. It is one of a number of medicines that can do so. Everything depends on the bigger picture—the rest of the story.

In virtually all injuries whether it be burns, sprains, fractures, torn ligaments or loss of consciousness homeopathy can play a vital, sometimes lifesaving, role.

thirty seven

Brown Recluse Spider Bite Treated with Lachesis

A three year old child, bitten on her left forearm by a Brown Recluse spider, was hospitalized in New Mexico. She was lying on her back and not very responsive to any stimulation–verbal or touch. She had been unresponsive for many hours. Covered in perspiration, her temperature was 100.3°F.

The venom of the Brown Recluse is extremely toxic and causes a blackish ulcer to appear at the site of the bite. As the venom spreads outward it causes the blood to break down and purplish bruising to appear together with swelling. The patient can have fever and chills and, if unlucky, can become drowsy and even comatose.

This little girl had an IV in her good arm and was receiving both an antibiotic and steroids.

A medical student, who was studying homeopathy, was on the pediatric service at the time. He realized the antibiotic and steroids were not acting and thought that if the child worsened she could develop a generalized blood infection (septicemia) and might have to undergo disfiguring surgery, possibly even an amputation. As it was, the swelling had already extended from the forearm up to, and including, the shoulder.

After consulting with several other homeopaths, he decided on *Lachesis,* prepared from the venom of the Bushmaster snake, an important homeopathic medicine. Because he knew that none of the doctors in the hospital would permit the use of homeopathic medicines, he placed a few drops of *Lachesis* in a syringe, added water, and, without being noticed, dripped some drops into her mouth.

Within ten minutes, the child suddenly woke up out of her semi-comatose state, stood up in the crib and started screaming bloody murder. She was crying for her mother and wanted to be picked up. *Lachesis* had so changed her energy that she had gone from a state of limpness and near lifelessness to a zesty, screaming girl. Before *Lachesis*, she had felt no pain. After *Lachesis*, she became very sensitive to pain.

Whenever a patient goes from a stuporous or dazed condition without pain, to one of alertness with pain, you can be sure they are improving. From then on, the child's wound began to heal. The swelling went down quickly, but the ulcer took several days to heal up. The rest of the hospitalization was uneventful and she was discharged.

thirty eight

Altitude Sickness Cured with Coca

Altitude sickness can be mild, moderate, severe, even fatal. Mild symptoms include:

- lack of appetite
- fatigue and weakness
- dizziness or lightheadedness
- sleepiness or sleeplessness
- shortness of breath on exertion
- rapid pulse
- and, less often, swelling of the hands, feet and face

As altitude sickness progresses, a dry cough, fever and shortness of breath at rest can occur. Sometimes, pulmonary edema (fluid in the lungs) can occur as well.

In the worst cases, the brain swells (cerebral edema) which, in turn, can cause a headache that does not respond to pain killers, balance problems, and gradual loss of consciousness. Retinal hemorrhage has been reported. With brain involvement, it is possible the person will die.

To protect against altitude sickness, people in the Andes Mountains in South America have chewed coca leaves and have done so for centuries. It is also a mild stimulant and can suppress hunger, thirst, fatigue, even pain. Though cocaine is extracted from coca leaves through complex chemical processes, coca leaf is not cocaine just as grapes are not wine. Coca leaves can be brewed and drunk as a tea or chewed. Coca leaf has also been made into a homeopathic medicine through dilution and succussion.

The following incident of altitude sickness concerned a forty-eight-year old man who had, the day before, returned to his home in Guatemala from Bolivia where he had been working in the high Andes.

The next morning his wife phoned one of my students, Patricia Osorio, to ask for her help. Her husband, she said, had been conducting a seminar for the previous five days at an altitude of over 4,000 meters. He was quite ill, she said. It so happened, I was teaching a workshop in Guatemala City that day so the students and I together took the case.

In addition to great fatigue, he had no appetite except for sweets. The night before, at 11 p.m. he suffered a chill with nausea. He vomited a bit of white foamy material and complained of a severe headache in the back of his head and temples. He was anxious and restless, tossing and turning. He awoke again at 3:30 a.m. with a chill and vomiting. His wife mentioned he had been under quite a lot of stress for the previous month.

At daybreak, he woke feeling very cold and did not want to get out of bed. "It is our ten-year-old daughter's birthday today," said his wife, "and a piñata is planned for the afternoon. I don't think my husband is going to be able to make it."

Homeopathic *Coca* is effective for the following symptoms, all of which he suffered from:

- Headache at high altitudes.
- Weakness at high altitudes.
- Headache with pain in the occiput and temples.
- Headache with chill.
- Lack of appetite yet wants sweets.
- Sleepiness with weariness.

He received a single dose of *Coca* 200c at midday. Three hours later, he got up, attended his daughter's birthday party and ate two sandwiches. *Coca* was not repeated. He was fine. Later, he told Patricia that during the night when he was so ill, he had great difficulty breathing. He did not mention this to his wife so as not to worry her. As might be expected, homeopathic *Coca* is known to produce and take away dyspnea (difficult breathing) at high altitudes which is worse at night.

Medical references to high altitude sickness suggest the first measure is to descend to a lower altitude. Our patient had already descended. In fact, that was when his symptoms began. Conventional treatment includes acetazolamide (Diamox) but that is usually suggested before and during ascent as it acts biochemically to increase oxygen in the blood. It is not very useful once altitude sickness has begun. Other measures are breathing oxygen, the drug, nifedipine, for acute pulmonary edema (fluid in the lungs) and the potent steroid, dexamethasone, should cerebral edema (swelling of the brain) occur. All measures employed by conventional medicine are palliative, take time to work, and have associated adverse effects.

Clearly, homeopathic *Coca* deserves to be in every mountain climber's backpack. It is noteworthy that chewing the coca leaves and taking homeopathic *Coca* have similar beneficial effects when in high altitudes. Interestingly, the homeopathic preparation can often have quite different effects from the crude substance.

Coca is known among homeopaths as a "small" medicine meaning that it is used infrequently. When it is prescribed, usually for the adverse effects of being in the high mountains, it can be extraordinarily useful.

thirty nine

End of Life - A Story of Transformation

Chaim was very close to death when I saw him in his daughter's home. She had begged me to come as he was far too ill to travel even the few miles from his house to my office. Chaim was seventy-eight and suffering from end-stage pancreatic cancer.

As I entered the bedroom I saw a gaunt and wasted man. I greeted him. "How are you?" I asked.

"I am one hundred percent perfect," he replied, without hesitating and with an air of certainty I found remarkable.

His daughter, Eliora, added, "He has been saying he is fine for five or six days now."

"What else does he say?" I asked, knowing that a patient's words could reveal their inner state *and* show the way to the appropriate homeopathic medicine.

"He says, 'Leave me alone,' and, 'Please, don't talk to me.'"

"Tell me about his behavior."

"From eleven till three in the afternoon he fights with me. He won't eat. I do everything I know to offer him food he likes but he refuses it. Sometimes he asks me to move him in bed. He is too weak to turn himself."

I learned from Eliora he was passing stool that was pale brown and had been odorless though it had a slight odor recently. His urine was dark brown and cloudy. He preferred to lie on his left side. His mouth, left arm and left inner thigh trembled from time to time. He was dehydrated, common, toward the end of life, and his mouth was dry. When he did drink, which was infrequently, he took little sips.

He was on a narcotic to control the pain.

"How was he before he started the narcotic?" I asked.

"He woke every night at three a.m.," she said. I made a note of the time. If a patient wakes regularly at the same hour, it can be a useful symptom.

Eliora's greatest concern was that her father should eat. In her distress, she went on and on about how he needed to eat. "He pushes me away when I offer him food," she said. "He gets angry."

I suggested that—by not eating—Chaim was allowing his body to shut down, dimming the lights as it were, and getting ready to die. "He knows what he is doing," I said. "It is an intelligent response to his situation."

I could see Eliora was unconvinced.

What to do? Chaim was fast approaching death and doing so in his own feisty way. I respected that. But Eliora wanted something else for her father. She hated fighting with him every day and his constant rejection of her was hard for her.

I knew his pancreatic cancer had already won—that it was a matter of a few days. But perhaps, I thought, Chaim's behavior contained a coded message and if I could break the code I would find a homeopathic medicine that could ease his final days.

In the homeopathic interview, often the first words the patient says contain a vital clue. Chaim's first words, "I am one hundred percent perfect," could not have been further off the mark. He might have said, "I'm fine, thank you," and I would have paid no attention. He could have said, "I'm dying," and that, too, would have struck me as reasonable. But no, he was, "One hundred percent perfect."

Knowing how rich our homeopathic literature is in unusual symptoms, I started to search. And there it was. In the Repertory, in the mind section, I read, "Says he is well when very sick." The rubric contained twenty-three medicines.

I then thought about how daily he fought with his daughter, refusing to eat. It was not his lack of appetite, common in advanced cancer, or even his refusal to eat, that intrigued me. It was that he got angry when Eliora tried to feed him. I turned to the Repertory again and read, "Anger when obliged to eat." There was only one entry, *Arsenicum album,* which also appeared in the previous rubric.

Arsenic is also known to have odorless stools, brown urine, and a tendency to take tiny sips of water. The repertorization:

- Mind, says he is well when very sick.
- Mind, anger, when obliged to eat.
- Stool, odorless.
- Urine, brown.
- Thirst for small quantities.
- Sleep, waking at 3 a.m.

Most patients needing *Arsenicum* are anxious, some to the point of anguish, and insist on someone being close by. Chaim was not in that *Arsenicum* state. But because *Arsenicum* did cover all his very striking symptoms, I prescribed it. I instructed Eliora to give him *Arsenicum album* 30c in water three times a day. That was July 16, 2008. I spoke with her two days later.

"I gave him three doses yesterday," she said, "and yesterday evening he wanted to get up...this after twenty-four hours of his not wanting to eat or drink. I got him up. He wanted to shower and I helped him take one. Before your medicine he wanted to do absolutely nothing. Also, last night he asked for carrot juice and drank it. This morning he ate half a pear. Then he said he wanted to rearrange the room! So I cleaned the room, changed the sheets, and moved the bed.

"And you know Dr. Robinson, yesterday he said, 'Don't abandon me,' and today he said, 'Don't forget me.' I am so happy. Thank you."

Chaim died July 23, 2008.

An orthodox Jew, Chaim was buried in Israel, according to Jewish custom.

Nine months later, Eliora came by the office to thank me. We spoke of her father's last days.

"Eliora," I said, "you seemed so happy after your father received *Arsenicum* even though he was dying."

"Yes," she said. "He was talking. He was able to connect. Before the *Arsenicum*, it was always me trying to connect with him. After, he connected with me."

At the beginning of life—infantile colic—at the end of life—on the deathbed, homeopathy eases us on.

forty

The Follow Up

The hardest part of being a doctor is not making the diagnosis, nor is it in prescribing medicines. It is evaluating the patient's progress, or lack thereof, during the follow up visits. Knowing if the patient is truly getting better is an art and science unto itself that is, unfortunately, neglected in the education of physicians. To know the patient is on the path to heath is more than seeing symptoms disappear, and more than having blood chemistries normalize. This chapter will explore this little discussed and most critical area of medicine.

HOW TO KNOW IF THE PATIENT IS IMPROVING, REMAINING THE SAME, OR WORSENING

Everyone who goes to a healthcare practitioner has the same goal–to feel better. What could be simpler? If you feel better, ipso facto, you are better. No matter the therapy (psychotherapy, allopathic drugs, homeopathic medicines, a better diet, an exercise regimen), if, after starting it, you feel better then that therapy is working.

Or is it?

Let's say I prescribe a homeopathic medicine for a depressed person who is unemployed. He comes back a month later, no longer depressed. In the meantime, he has found a good paying job that he likes. Was it my homeopathic medicine or the job? I, personally, would vote for the job.

Let's say the allopath starts a patient on an anti-hypertensive for high blood pressure. Six weeks later, the pressure is normal. But in that same period, the patient began a rigorous diet and lost fifteen pounds. He looks better and he is proud of himself. What is responsible for the better blood pressure? I'd vote for the weight loss. Of course, the only way to be sure would be to stop the anti-hypertensive and check the BP.

Let's say I prescribe homeopathy for a person with low energy, depression, and total body aches. She comes back a month later looking radiant. "I feel so much better," she says. No depression, great energy, and no aches and pains. But in that month, she started an exercise program, lost some weight and fell in love. What gets the credit? One cannot know for sure. What very well may have happened is the homeopathic medicine so changed her outlook and energy that she was able to lose weight, exercise and fall in love or it could have been all due to her lifestyle changes. She feels empowered, that she is the author of her better life, and that is the most important thing.

A child has a fever of 104°F. I give a homeopathic medicine at 4 p.m. The following morning he is afebrile. Shall I give homeopathy the credit? Perhaps yes, perhaps no. The human body is perfectly capable of conquering a fever in twelve hours with no help from homeopathy, allopathy or anything else. So the answer is homeopathy may have acted but may not have. But, if the temperature falls from 104°F to 99.5° F within twenty minutes of taking the homeopathic medicine *and* the child falls into a peaceful sleep after having been delirious with his high fever *and* awakes the next morning with no fever, good energy *and* an appetite, well then, yes, the homeopathic medicine probably acted.

In this last case, the criterion is that **the treatment shall have interrupted and changed the usual, expected course of the illness in a dramatic and favorable way**. So, in addition to the fever dropping quickly to near normal, the delirium ceasing, the sleep becoming peaceful, the energy and the appetite returned.

Let's say a small child, under age five, has otitis media (middle ear infection). The pediatrician gives an antibiotic and the infection clears. A definite cure. But wait a moment. Ten days later, the child develops another ear infection. A different antibiotic is prescribed. The child recovers. Another cure? Well, let's wait and see. Sure enough, two weeks later the child develops a third ear infection requiring yet a third antibiotic. This scenario is replayed for four months. With the coming of spring, there is no more otitis media. But the following winter, the otitis starts up again with more antibiotics, brief periods of improvement and more relapses—a therapeutic quandary seen hundreds of times in every pediatrician's office. Every time the child has a bacterial infection, the antibiotic selected is proven in the petri dish to kill that bacterium; it is given *and* it acts, but then the otitis reoccurs. What is going on? Obviously, the child's immune system is not up to par. The child's parents bring him to a homeopath who, after a lengthy period of questioning the parents and observing the child, gives a single homeopathic medicine that corresponds (as I have said repeatedly) to the nature of the child *and* the peculiar aspects of the otitis. No more otitis. Five years later, the mother sees the homeopath about another matter and says, "After you treated Sunny five years ago he never had another ear infection." Coincidence? Homeopaths don't think so. We believe the homeopathic medicine acted curatively, stimulating the immune system to function normally and the improved immune system kept the child healthy. Can the homeopath prove the homeopathic medicine was responsible? No. But the circumstantial evidence is convincing especially when similar successful outcomes occur repeatedly with many children.

Many sick persons present with a complicated array of symptoms affecting many systems and organs and when some problems improve and others do not it can be daunting—trying to understand if, overall, the patient's health is improving.

Let's look at some examples.

A teenage girl had frequent asthma attacks every week. Her asthma began in childhood. She was on two inhalers which allowed her to function. After six months of homeopathic treatment, the asthma attacks ceased and she got off her allopathic meds. Everyone–the girl, her parents, and the homeopath–were delighted. However, a year later, she had a violent asthma attack requiring hospitalization. This was **not** a good result. Best if she had had milder and milder attacks further and further apart and then none. The idea is to **strengthen the patient and not the disease**. With proper treatment, she would have been less and less sensitive to allergens. When her asthma did return, however, it was stronger than ever. Though she had a grace period of a year, the fact that the asthma returned requiring hospitalization suggested the homeopathic medicine was not correct.

In the past year I treated a woman with arthritic pains. A month later, those pains had diminished considerably. Though she was quite pleased, I asked her how she was feeling in general and she said she had little desire to do anything and was still very, very sad about the passing of her father a year earlier. Not a good result. We **always** want to see an improvement in the general energy and outlook and then, later, an improvement in the physical problems, in her case, arthritic pains. So, I changed her medicine, the pains returned but her mood and energy improved. Later, her pains began to diminish.

One can see the homeopath's expectations are far different from the allopath's. For the latter, if the arthritic pains diminish that is all he cares about. The patient's stamina and outlook are of slight concern.

As a patient improves his **interest in his daily activities returns**. So, the child recovering from a high fever, no longer wants to be held or carried non-stop by his mother and, instead, starts crawling about the floor, interested in his toys.

A low energy patient (with whatever physical complaints) will report, after a successful homeopathic prescription, "I'm doing more around the house. I'm out in the garden again," or "I've started exercising again," etc. The negative corollary is when the migraines (or whatever physical complaint) have diminished but there is no joy in life. It means, **the wrong medicine has been given** and the homeopath must re-take the case as if for the first time, i.e., with a fresh and open mind looking for a medicine that more closely corresponds not only to the complaints but to the person.

To recapitulate: in a curative response the patient will have:

- Greater energy.
- Renewed interest in his daily activities.
- A more positive outlook.

Think of Chaim (Chapter Thirty-eight). Even though close to death, after receiving *Arsenicum album*, he wanted to shower, to eat and drink a bit, and re-arrange the room! *And* he connected emotionally with his daughter.

Or, my hospitalized patient with pneumonia (Chapter Twenty-eight). After *Phosphorus*, not only did the cough, fever and chill disappear, but her energy soared. "I'm walking around. I'm ready to go," she said with animation.

THE LAW OF CURE

Homeopaths are fortunate to have a set of rules for evaluating their patients' progress or lack thereof. It is known as the **Law of Cure** and was formulated by Constantine Hering (1800 to 1880). Born in Germany, he emigrated to the United States in the 1830's. After observing thousands of successful recoveries with homeopathic medicines, he concluded that healing occurred in a consistent pattern.

Firstly, a cure must begin at the deepest level, that of the mind and the emotions, and from there proceed from more vital organs outwards to less and less vital organs, eventually to the extremities and skin.

Secondly, as the body heals itself, symptoms will appear and disappear in the reverse chronology of their original appearance.

Thirdly, healing progresses from the uppermost part of the body gradually moving downwards.

Often Hering's Law is abbreviated and the order changed as follows:

- From above downwards.
- From inside outwards, or, in other words, from the center to the periphery.
- In the reverse order of the appearance of the symptoms.

So, in the autoimmune disease known as **vitiligo**, there is a deficiency of melanocytes resulting in depigmentation of the skin causing white patches to appear. Vitiligo is more common in the subcontinent than in the U.S. and I have seen numerous patients in India with vitilgo cured with homeopathy. The interesting point is that the white patches must repigment from above downward. If there are white lesions on the face and arms, those on the face must disappear first and **those on the upper part of the face before those lower on the face**. At the same time that the facial patches are repigmenting, it is quite possible that increased white patches may appear on the arms. As the law "from above downwards" is operative, it is okay. Those lesions on the arms will eventually disappear without repeating the homeopathic medicine. When the patches of vitiligo increase on the arms, the patient will protest loudly, "But look, doctor, it is so much worse on my arms." The homeopath who abides by the Law of Cure will reassure his patient that everything is in order and that, eventually (months), the vitiligo will also go from the arms and hands.

In one of many trips to study with Dr. Prafull Vijayakar, an outstanding homeopath in Mumbai, India, I saw him rigorously apply this law. If the lesions disappeared on lower areas but not the ones higher up, he always changed the homeopathic medicine, saying the improvement was not according to the Law of Cure and therefore would not be permanent.

If a patient has psoriasis involving the scalp, the topmost part of the scalp should clear first and then clear outward and downward all over the head. Afterwards, the upper trunk and upper extremities must clear followed by the lower extremities.

The same order will be seen in a successful prescription for arthritic pains. First the cervical spine must improve, then the shoulders, elbows, wrists, and hands followed by the lower back, hips, knees, ankles and feet.

Though the patient may complain loudly about the remaining pains lower down, as long as the upper pains are better, the patient is headed for cure.

I once treated a man with debilitating sciatic pain. Three months after beginning homeopathic treatment, the sciatic pain was mostly gone but there was a new pain a bit higher up the back. I knew immediately the Law of Cure had been contravened, retook the case and re-prescribed. On the new medicine, all complaints resolved.

Hering insisted that more vital organs improve before less vital ones. This concept is nicely illustrated in the case of a desperately ill woman that was reported by the Indian homeopath, Dr. Narendra Mehta, in his book, *The Follow-Up*. Mehta described a seventy-one-year-old woman in coma following a stroke in the right side of the brain leaving her paralyzed on the left side of her body. He took a careful history and prescribed *Arsenicum album* 200c, a single dose. The following day she was able to obey simple commands and sit up for two minutes without support. Four days later, the patient's son rang Mehta in alarm saying that his mother's face was grossly swollen and she could not open her eyes. He visited her and found she could sit without support and talk and recognize everyone. Indeed, her face was swollen and bloated, but her level of consciousness was greatly improved as was her ability to sit. Because her level of consciousness had improved, Mehta inferred that the brain, heretofore swollen rendering her unconscious was no longer as swollen and that, in all likelihood, the swelling had moved outward to her face–a positive sign. He administered placebo. Two days later, she complained of joint pains which she had had earlier in her life. In accordance with Hering's law, this was a return of an old symptom and a good sign. Her face was more swollen. Again, placebo was given. She continued to improve. Twenty days after the only dose of *Arsenicum* she was sitting, talking and laughing. Five weeks after *Arsenicum* she developed an abscess on the head. Mehta knew it was a good development because the illness had now exteriorized to the skin. No antibiotics were given. The patient continued to a full recovery.

The woman's journey from coma and left-sided paralysis was a dramatic example of Hering's Law of Cure. She went from coma to greater and greater awareness followed by joint pain, an old problem. Then, as she continued to improve, the abscess of the scalp appeared. By seventh week the abscess had healed and she was walking unaided.

This most dramatic cure occurred in India, a country where hundreds of millions of people know about homeopathy and use it. It is cited here to give an idea of just how powerful homeopathic medicines can be when correctly prescribed.

forty one

In this chapter, we take a look at two relatively new homeopathic medicines that promise to be of use, possibly great use, in this nuclear age.

Radiation Sickness.

How Homeopathy Can Help.

An Irish (True) Tale.

Part I

For more than thirty-five years homeopathy has been the central passion of my life. I have studied with renowned homeopaths from many countries. The work of Nuala Eising, an Irish homeopath whom I count as a friend as well as colleague, stands out for its originality and usefulness. In the fascinating account that follows, it appears that two substances she proved, *Granite* and *Marble*, may well prove to be of major importance in the treatment of radiation sickness. Though news from Chernobyl has faded, the toxic radiation will be around for thousands of years.

Ihor Gramotkin, director of the Chernobyl power plant, was asked when the reactor site would again be habitable, he replied, "At least 20,000 years." (Time Magazine, April 26, 2011)

And then came the Fukushima nuclear disaster on March 11, 2011 with its release of Cesium-134 (half-life 2.1 years), Cesium -137 (half-life

30 years), Iodine-131 (half-life 8 days), and Strontium-90 (half-life 28.8 years). Depending on what source you read, the adverse health effects of the Fukushima spill range from minimal to catastrophic. The purpose of this small essay is not to enter that debate but to show how homeopathic *Granite* and *Marble* may be quite useful in countering radiation sickness.

In 1993, Nuala Eising gained first-hand experience in observing and treating the effects of radiation sickness by living with and treating a small group of children from Belarus, an area particularly hard hit by fallout from the Chernobyl spill, April 26, 1986. What Nuala discovered was that these children had been strangely affected by growing up in a radioactive fallout zone. Though they did not have thyroid cancer or leukemia, their intellectual, emotional and physical makeup was drastically altered presumably by years of being exposed to radioactive elements. Homeopathy restored these children to health.

But before discussing the condition of the Belarus children prior to and after homeopathic treatment, one must begin at the beginning, with the captivating tale of how Nuala came to learn that homeopathic *Granite* and homeopathic *Marble* were key medicines in the treatment of radiation sickness.

For years, Nuala had had prophetic dreams, dreams in which she was guided to discover new homeopathic medicines, some of which are on track to become homeopathic medicines of major importance. She learned about granite as a homeopathic medicine via two dreams in November, 1984. Prior to the dreams she knew nothing whatsoever about granite other than it was a rock common to parts of Ireland. The first dream took place in Connemara, a bleak, rocky, mountainous area in the far west of Ireland. From Galway, one heads west a few miles before finding Connemara.

In the first dream, Nuala found herself looking at a picture of Connemara with its hills, bleak and grey. Over the picture were the words:

CONNEMARA IS THE DAY AFTER.

Then appeared five more pictures, each one of a person from Connemara in a wooden frame. There was a caption above each picture:

CONNEMARA PEOPLE ARE INTROVERTED.

CONNEMARA PEOPLE ARE INCESTUOUS.

CONNEMARA PEOPLE ARE MORE PRONE TO CANCER THAN ANYWHERE ELSE IN THE COUNTRY.

CONNEMARA PEOPLE HAVE MORE DOWNS SYNDROME CHILDREN THAN ANYWHERE ELSE IN THE COUNTRY.

CONNEMARA PEOPLE ARE TALLER ON AVERAGE THAN ANYWHERE ELSE IN THE COUNTRY. THEY HAVE IN FACT GROWN LIKE CANCER.

These five pictures with captions were followed in the same dream with a question and answer:

WHAT HAVE CONNEMARA PEOPLE GOT IN COMMON? GRANITE.

THE SECOND DREAM IN NUALA'S WORDS

I am looking out of the window. In the sky I see a white dot. This I know to be Granite as a homeopathic remedy. As I look at the dot, it explodes, becoming a piece of beautiful white lace. Slowly, it moves through the atmosphere, changing shape as it moves. It takes on the shape of butterflies and birds, always remaining as white lace. When it has moved through the whole atmosphere it drops to the ground in front of me. I look down – it is a white dove, dead because it has cleared the atmosphere of radioactivity.

The dreams set Nuala in motion. She contacted a geologist friend at University College, Galway, and learned that Connemara granite has one of the highest levels of radioactivity of all the granites found in Ireland and Britain. Connemara granite contains three radioactive elements:

Potassium	3-4% by weight	alpha rays
Uranium	1-10 ppm	alpha, beta and gamma rays
Thorium	10-50 ppm	alpha, beta, and gamma rays

She also learned that, indeed, Connemara, did have a higher level of cancer and Downs Syndrome than the rest of Ireland. Also, Connemara people tended to be introverted and there was said to be a lot of inbreeding in Connemara. Her impression was they seemed large.

Nuala took a piece of this granite and had it potentized to the 30c potency with which she did a proving. Fifteen people, eight women and seven men, ranging in ages from twenty to forty years, took the *Granite* 30c. None of them knew what they were taking. They lived in various parts of Ireland. Each of them wrote down all symptoms: mental, emotional, physical, sleep, dreams–everything they noticed. Each took the *Granite* 30c three times a day with instructions to stop as soon as definite symptoms appeared.

The complete proving of *Granite* 30c along with *Marble* 30c can be found in the booklet, *The Provings of Granite, Marble and Limestone* by Nuala Eising, The Burren School of Homeopathy, Caherawoneen, Kinvara, Co. Galway, Ireland. Unfortunately, the booklet is now out of print. (The Burren School was closed in 2006.)

In an interview with Nuala, spanning several hours, she mentioned aspects of the provings. "Many of the provers became suspicious of friends coming round to visit," she said. "They were of the mind set, 'What do they want from me now?'" This lead to a new rubric, "Delusions: he will be dispossessed."

One prover wrote that she had a, "Leave me alone," and "Don't come near me," feeling. One prover noted that she found herself sitting, "With arms folded tight – trying to keep everything in."

Nuala told me that, sometime after completing the proving of *Granite,* she and Misha Norland, noted British homeopath, once stopped for tea at a pub in Connemara.

"The owner served us. He had his arms folded in front of him and he walked up and down the room, never once took his eyes off us. He kept his eyes on us the whole time.

"Connemara people stare at you," she continued. "They are very suspicious of strangers and keep an eye on them."

Back to the proving.

One prover wrote that he felt, "a profound feeling of introversion – of not wanting to be around people and give them any of my space."

"Don't touch me," was another comment.

Another wrote of having become, "very anti-social – to the extent that at work I chose to do the pieces of work that entailed not being in contact with people."

Another found herself needing to leave when she had visitors.

Another spoke of being, "full of negativity." Another noticed, "a deep feeling of sadness and worthlessness."

Another felt, "a lot of hatred for all those meaningless people who seemed to keep invading my space." She noticed she was, "very insolent and rude."

One woman said she felt she was fighting all the time, "for my own territory."

Another said she felt, "very suspicious of the motives of others, including friends."

Another: "I am feeling close to no-one."

Another: "I feel contempt for others – they seemed so worthless and insignificant."

After the proving concluded, Nuala got some interesting feedback from friends and family of the provers. One comment: "He was unbearable to be with." Another said, "I couldn't stand being around him."

One husband told of his despair because his wife was so withdrawn and cold. Another husband went so far as to temporarily leave, "because of my wife's bluntness and anger."

Out of the proving came these rubrics:

- Delusions: people seem mentally and physically inferior.
- Delusions: of being attacked.
- Delusions: one's space is being invaded. Censorious, critical.
- Aversion to being approached.
- Contemptuous.
- Dictatorial.
- Estranged from friends.
- Indifference to everything.
- Malicious.
- Quarrelsome.
- Reproaches others.
- Rudeness.

- Selfish.
- Snappish.
- Spoken to, aversion to being.
- Suspicious.
- Unfeeling.
- Unsympathetic.

One can see from the proving that *Granite* produced a state of profound introversion, suspiciousness, a dislike of people (including family and friends) and a desire to be left totally alone. When with people, they behaved rudely even hatefully and maliciously and were often quarrelsome.

In addition to the mental and emotional symptoms, a number of provers, all men, experienced flu-like symptoms: headaches, sore throats, high fevers (103°F), limbs heavy and aching, much sweating and weakness. One man reported waking at 3 a.m. with a headache, sore throat and swollen glands. The joints ached and felt heavy and he felt very cold. By noon his temperature reached 103°F. By 9 p.m. he was completely delirious. The fever did not break until 4 a.m. the next day. The swollen glands and sore throat kept on for four days.

When I visited Nuala in her home in Kinvara in 2011, she told how within ten to fourteen days of the blowout at Chernobyl, when radiation levels were at their highest, a flu-like syndrome appeared among those exposed. Years later, when she was re-reading the proving, it struck her that homeopathic *Granite* had produced many symptoms typical of flu, especially the exhaustion and general achiness.

It may be hard to accept that a tiny piece of granite diluted 10^{-60} (Yes, that's a fraction with 60 zeros in the denominator!) could produce such violent flu-like symptoms. But it did, not only in that one man, but in several other male provers. When a substance is potentized, that is, diluted and succussed many times, it then has the power to disrupt the Vital Force in such a way that hundreds of striking symptoms are produced in both the mind and the body.

It was not until nine years later that Nuala came to use homeopathic *Granite* in the treatment of radiation sickness.

Part II

In 1993, Nuala was invited to work with a group of twelve children from Gomel, Belarus, some 40 kilometers from Chernobyl, who had come to Ireland primarily for homeopathic treatment. The children ranged in age from nine to eleven. Though they did not have thyroid cancer or leukemia, they were very definitely different from any children Nuala had encountered. They had lived amidst significant levels of radioactivity for seven years.

It was the beginning of November, 1993, when Nuala met them. She reported, "The most noticeable thing about the children was their sadness and sense of resignation." It was not only their manner but how they looked. "They were very pale and translucent in appearance. They were also very 'wide-eyed' – looking directly and very seriously. Their fear of being touched was also very apparent. All of us who met the children at this stage were mesmerized by them. We felt that we would do anything for these children."

At that point, Nuala had no clear idea that these children would need homeopathic *Granite.* She planned to interview the children in the usual homeopathic fashion expecting that each would need a different medicine, based on their constitution. It did not turn out that way.

Immediately after meeting the children, Nuala had a dream in which a man, who had been in her dreams for years, came up behind her left shoulder. Apparently, this particular, very helpful man, always came up behind her left shoulder. He started to lecture:

> *The children from Belarus will need Granite first, but then they must have Marble. Granite is always appropriate for the initial and peripheral effects of radioactivity. These children have undergone a metamorphosis. Look at Limestone and Marble. They are both calcium carbonate. The intense heat and pressure when Granite is forming turns Limestone to Marble. Although Marble is calcium, it is metamorphic calcium. When people are close to a major radioactive disaster like Chernobyl, there is at first an intense internal heat, and gradually their calcium cells begin to change. These children are the metamorphic version of their original state, and as such, they need*

Marble, which is the most similar. Look at the children, their pallor, their translucence—just like white marble. Marble crumbles from the inside—the shine on the outside holds it together. The same happens to people affected by high levels of radiation—they disintegrate from the inside.

That dream occurred in November, 1993. Nuala had had an earlier dream, in 1992, when the same man appeared (again behind her left shoulder) and told her to go to the Inagh Valley. He was very specific. "Make sure you go to the Inagh Valley in Connemara, not in Co. Clare." He showed her a valley with a big river running through it with mountains on one side and a road on the other. "What you are looking for," he said, "is to be found in the hills on the other side of the river." He then showed Nuala pictures of people living in that valley. She thought they seemed "wild and lawless."

She went to the valley a number of times, not knowing what it was she was looking for. Eventually, she decided simply to wait, trusting that something would turn up. One day a student in Nuala's school of homeopathy told her a dream in which Nuala took her to some place in Connemara where the student proceeded to get crushed under a large, white rock. It quite freaked her out and she asked Nuala, (in the dream) what to do. Nuala told her she was undergoing a metamorphosis and not to worry.

Nuala wrote, "When she told me about this dream, I realized that the rock had to be marble or quartz, being the only white rocks in the area."

Some months later, Nuala and a student were sitting around a fire one night after a couple of drinks. The student said to Nuala, "I can't understand your stamina. You must be on something. You must be on marble." Afterwards, the student hadn't a clue why she had said it. Nuala tucked the incident away and continued to wait.

After the second dream, that occurred the night after meeting the Belarus children, she knew she must prove marble. It was not so easy. Most of the rocks she and a friend picked up were quartz. Eventually, they were directed to an old man. When they went to his house they were met at the door by a gorgeous white cat. The old man invited them in for tea but was rude and suspicious. Nuala wrote, "He exuded the aura of, 'These people are trying to get something for nothing,'" After much explaining that they did not want a large quantity of marble the man finally gave them a small piece. Nuala handed him £10 and he offered change. Nuala told to him to keep it, that they had caused him a lot of trouble and they wanted him to enjoy a few pints. "The atmosphere changed immediately," she wrote, "and he became very friendly. He invited us to call on him anytime we wanted more marble."

She added, "The man was, I was aware, living on granite," a reference to the proving she had done of *Granite.*

This proving was made with the 30c potency of *Marble.* There were ten provers, six females, four males. Each was instructed to take one dose three times a day until symptoms appeared and then stop. Some provers had immediate symptoms the first day and stopped. Others took *Marble* 30c for up to five days before symptoms appeared.

Perhaps the most striking theme of the *Marble proving* was how cat-like the provers felt. Some "cat" comments from different provers:

- *I wake at 4 a.m. I was purring and thought I was a cat. I was stretching and squirming in the bed thinking I am the most gorgeous creature that ever walked the planet. Everyone is going to love me, I am so charming.*

- *When I woke this morning, I felt very pleasant and relaxed and very aware of my body. My movement is slow and graceful. I remind myself of my cat and think I know how she feels.*

- *I wanted to curl up beside the fire all day. Would like someone to take care of all my needs.*

- *I'm like a cat that got the cream.*

- *I'm discovering the use of my body and my eyes. My eyes feel wide. I feel distinctly feline. I can use my body and eyes and people will do anything for me. Everyone wants to help and I love being taken care of. I'm aware that I look very honest and open and everyone is falling for it. I look in the mirror and see the beauty and charm that everyone else obviously must see. I think I'm a bit self-absorbed since starting the proving—but that feels fine.*

- *I looked in the mirror yesterday and thought how beautiful I am. I keep cutting my hair.*

- *When I look at myself in the mirror naked, I see nice curves and smooth skin (usually I feel ugly and see hairiness, spottiness and stretch marks). I glanced in the mirror and saw cat's eyes (which I had years ago). Also I'm extremely aware of birds. I have to stop and watch them when I walk or look for them if I hear them. I'm singing all the time.*

- *I should be a princess in some exotic warm country. Quiet and refined, with lots of people taking care of my needs—quietly, discreetly.*

- *I feel like a newly born kitten that hasn't opened its eyes.*

- *I've imagined myself on a roof, jumping off and landing softly on my feet. I've thought about jumping from heights a few times during the proving. I wouldn't like to jump into water.*

- *I get a great desire to curl up beside my husband and be stroked. It has to be when I want to—not the other way around*

- *I've brushed my hair more frequently and stroke and play with my hair. I'm using my nose more, smelling things and I seem to twitch my nose about.*

- *I keep cutting and brushing my hair. I am concerned about the condition of my hair. I keep looking for split ends and trimming them and brushing my hair. I spend hours doing this.*

- *I have this whole thing about hair. I want to remove it from my body. I used hair remover for the first time in my life last week and I think I will use it again because the hair is coming back now (I used to scorn this kind of thing). Now I feel like it and want to do it while the feeling is there. There is a lovely, sexy feeling about having smooth, silky legs caressed.*

- *I'm noticing birds and looking for them. I saw a bird today. My mouth was open and I could feel what it would be like to scrunch into it.*

- *I've been thinking of growing my nails long and have become more aware of my teeth. This morning my four year old daughter woke me and asked me to scratch her with my claws. She then told me I was growing whiskers. I've also been fantasizing having sex with different men.*

- *I feel good near the sea. Want to take walks by the sea. Would like to go in, but the idea of getting cold and wet does not appeal. This has been going on throughout the proving.*

- *I went to England on the boat. I got very comfortable and sprawled out on a long seat (I wouldn't usually). I didn't like the look of the sea. Thought how awful it would be to get wet and cold.*

- *I noticed a real couldn't-care-about-anyone attitude. It's hard to describe. Like I'm so self-contained—why should I care about you?*

Some provers became risk takers and enjoyed frightening others.

- *I took my sister for a drive. I drove through a red light—she freaked out and I just laughed. Her husband was waiting at home and had asked me to let him know that she had been dropped off OK. I was supposed to go back and tell him, but I didn't I went out instead. I knew he would be worried, but I stayed out for a few hours. When I got to his house, he said he was worried (which I knew anyway). I just laughed. I'd played a game.*

- *I was driving into town with my daughter. I picked up a male hitchhiker. I had to overtake a very long truck and was not as cautious as normal. I had to do 90 mph to overtake it. While overtaking, I caught sight of my hitchhiker in the rear-view mirror. He was terrified, sitting on the edge of his seat. Suddenly, I was enjoying myself, grinning to myself and wondering if I could freak him out a bit more. When I let him off, I was looking around to see if I could find some more hitchhikers to freak out—I was enjoying playing cat and mouse.*

- *I keep forcing confrontation. I'm also being demanding, selfish. It's as though only what I want and how I feel is important.*

- This particular comment turned out to be characteristic of most of the Belarus children prior to being treated with homeopathy.

Part III

I asked Nuala to recollect her first impressions of the Belarus children.

"Well, they spoke no English. What struck me about the kids was how stationary and blocked they were. They were very tight. Visibly emotionless. They had a tendency to stare at you. They were all extremely pale. We had no medical history on them but presumably they were anemic. Their paleness had a translucence about it. They all had huge purplish and black circles halfway down their cheeks.

"They were all very tired and had no energy compared to the local (Irish) kids. They needed constant naps.

"I felt they were suspicious of us. We had a bit of a breakthrough when I asked them to teach me Russian. They got more animated.

"When they played with each other there was what I would call a cruel mischief going on. One day, one kid locked one of his companions in a room then flung the key into a field. We had to break down the door.

You could imagine a two or three year old doing that but not a ten year old.

"I can say they were intellectually quite bright, but emotionally stunted. They all played chess.

"Other Irish that lived and worked with these children—we all got the feeling that these kids were afraid that something awful was going to happen and that they had to be prepared for it."

One girl said to Nuala, "People in Belarus are all waiting for something terrible to happen. They lock themselves away in their flats and they do not say hello to anyone, including their neighbors."

The same girl reported a dream about a trip with her mother and not knowing where they were going. "I have two questions in my mind—why was I born and why do I have to live in this life."

The girl went on to describe where they lived. "We live on the 8th floor of a block of flats. There is a big window in the kitchen overlooking the city. Everything becomes smaller. I can make judgments and decisions. My mother comes in and says, 'Don't set yourself above others.' But I do." She then told Nuala she was too tired to talk more and excused herself. Nuala touched her on the shoulder and she recoiled. "She got quite freaked."

Another child had a dream about being a cosmonaut in space, going further and further into space and not knowing where he was going.

"Their fear of touch was very obvious. They withdrew—no—recoiled is a better word, when we attempted to touch them. Also, there was this haughtiness."

Though Nuala started out to take each child's case individually and search for the *simillimum*, she quickly noticed that virtually all their symptoms were alike. "I decided to treat them as though they were suffering from an epidemic, in this case, radiation poisoning," she said.

On a Friday evening in early November, *Granite* 30c was given to all the children on the basis of:

- The idea that something terrible was going to happen.
- The sense of invasion.
- Fear of people.
- Fear of touch.
- The haughty, disdainful manner suggestive of homeopathic *Platina* (made from the element platinum)

"On Monday I couldn't believe my eyes!" Nuala told me. "The kids were all waving and shouting, 'Nuala! Nuala!' They were all animated. The girls hugged me. They were smiling. The boys shook hands. It was like *Granite* had taken down a wall. The improvement continued. They became happier, less fearful, more 'huggy' and their energy increased."

Nuala and other homeopaths assumed that after *Granite*, the children would need *Phosphorus* (made from the element, phosphorus) but that did not turn out to be the case.

"As we lived with and got to know the children, it was apparent that they were very cold, both emotionally and physically. They were very self-centered, haughty and very selfish. They were demanding, but in a quiet manner. Everything was noiseless, including their 'huffs.' They were quite independent in that they would go off by themselves and play for hours. But if they wanted you or your attention, they wanted it NOW! They were extremely charming and very graceful in movement. The young Belarusian girl who stayed with us would come up to me, look into my eyes and say, 'I would like this or that,' and I would have no choice but to say yes. Or if I was giving attention to anyone, she would move quietly and gracefully in between and say, 'I do ballet for you now.' There was also a lot of deceit and spitefulness."

January arrived and Nuala was mulling over what homeopathic medicine to give to the young Belarusian girl. She was favoring *Platina* but it did not quite fit. Then one night, Nuala had a dream in which she saw three of the children standing in front of her. The same man came up behind her shoulder and said,

> *Nuala, look at these children. You were a cat when you were doing the Marble proving. These children are cats all the time. They need Marble and they need it now. The thing with Marble people is that they are likely to look like Phosphorus, be as arrogant as Platina and be as charming and deceitful as Thuja. While Platina may dazzle with possessions, name-dropping, etc., Marble will only do so with their eyes and bodies. These children need Marble now.*

The dream, with its message, coincided with what Nuala was observing. One of the Belarusian girls, Rivka, was staying with Nuala. "She was unbelievably selfish," Nuala told me. "It was like watching a cat. You know the way a cat will go off when they want and when they want to sit on your lap they will? Rivka was like that. If I started to pay attention to my daughter, Rivka would literally step in between us and look me straight in the eye—very seductively—and move her body, swaying seductively and say, 'I do ballet for you now.' She did this frequently. If I didn't let her dance right away, she'd huff and go off."

All the girls from Belarus were obsessed with having Barbie dolls. In Belarus, a Barbie cost the equivalent of what a doctor earned in a week. "When we took them to toy stores," said Nuala, "all the girls wanted Barbie dolls and all the boys wanted windup toys. When they did get something, they put it away and NEVER shared."

Rivka was always taking from my daughter. I got curious and visited the other families with Belarus children and I heard the same thing everywhere—total selfishness. They were completely unhelpful. They avoided chores. One man in our village reported that when he gave attention to his son, the Belarus boy living with them could not tolerate it.

One day Nuala's oldest daughter took two Belarusian girls and Nuala's youngest daughter, Zoe, swimming. Only the young Belarusian girl knew how to swim. "She persuaded Zoe to go into the big pool with her. She pulled my daughter into the deep part of the pool. Zoe nearly drowned and had to be rescued. When they got home, Zoe freaked and had difficulty breathing. I gave her *Aconite* and was sitting beside her on the couch comforting her."

Rivka came over to Nuala several times, attempting to get Nuala's attention away from Zoe. At one point, she literally placed herself between Nuala and Zoe and said, "I do ballet for you now."

"No, not right now. Zoe needs me," said Nuala, firmly. Rivka went off in a huff. "I was pissed off but the homeopathy side of me was very interested. 'Wow!' I thought. 'This is as cold as you can get.'"

That was the tipping point. Although she had begun the proving of *Marble,* it was not complete. Nevertheless, she decided then and there to give Rivka *Marble* 30c. She talked to other families with Belarus children and heard stories of similar behavior. "In the end I gave *Marble* to all but two of the children. These two I gave *Medorrhinum.* They were hyper-energetic, passionate about the sea and loved heavy metal music. I could imagine them (culture allowing) wearing earrings and chains, etc."

After receiving *Marble,* the children made significant gains. The extreme rings under the eyes started to disappear. "Day by day, you could see them recede," said Nuala. "The two boys who got *Medorrhinum*—their circles did not go away.

"Amazing changes occurred on the emotional level. Their selfishness melted away. They started to open up. The kids started to share. They became more helpful. They helped with the chores. Two days after receiving *Marble*, one boy came up behind me and put his arms around me and said, 'I'm so happy. I have a second mom.'"

As mentioned, when Nuala first prescribed *Marble* to Rivka, she had not yet completed the proving of *Marble*. As results from the *Marble* proving came in she noted the cat theme was quite prominent and then realized that the Belarus children, prior to receiving homeopathic *Marble*, had, in fact, been acting very cat-like.

The two boys who got *Medorrhinum* did not improve. Two weeks before all the children were to return to Belarus, Nuala gave *Marble* to them. "They also did very well on it," wrote Nuala. "By the time they left in April, the children were all very healthy, energetic, loving and caring. Just before they left, I asked them what they would remember about Ireland. They said, 'The love.' That was wonderful to hear because just after Christmas I had asked them the same question and they all mentioned the things they had got."

Though the children returned home, Nuala continued to follow them for five years. Once a year she travelled to Belarus and once a year the same children returned to Ireland. During the first two years, Nuala repeated *Marble* with some of the children when necessary. "After two years, I knew that *Granite* and *Marble* had worked as by that time I could see their individual constitutions and neither *Granite* nor *Marble* were needed."

"During one trip to Belarus, a female Russian doctor gave everyone in a village *Granite* and they all got better."

During two different trips to Belarus, Nuala got quite ill. "A Belarus doctor with a Geiger counter was showing us a village that had been evacuated and was deserted. The levels of radioactivity were very high."

"I was extremely exhausted and had diarrhea," she recalled. "I wanted to be left alone. When I realized I was sick from radiation I took one little tablet of *Granite* 30c. I felt better within hours.

There were unplanned controls. The adults that were in charge of the Belarus children had two children of their own. They did not want their children treated as they lived outside the Gomel area and did not consider they had been affected by radiation.

"Their two children were initially in better shape than the twelve children from Gomel," said Nuala. "At the time of leaving, the two who had not been treated were excessively pale, lacking in stamina, serious and withdrawn. To my mind, this proved that the fresh air and good food were not the only factors in the change which was so remarkable in the twelve children."

Nuala did mention to me that *Granite* can be used to offset the harmful effects of radiation therapy, often prescribed in cancer. A single dose of *Granite* 30c should suffice.

Part III

The Genius of Homeopathy

Genius

here refers to the prevailing spirit and distinctive character of homeopathy. With its unique concepts and inclusive methodology, homeopathy is the only medicine that addresses subjective and objective symptoms at the same time. Both the invisible sensations and feelings that reside within every patient and the measurable, quantitative data that our senses and instruments register—both are fully recognized, valued and utilized in the practice of homeopathy.

forty two

Here The Genius Of Homeopathy Is On Display As A Series Of Medicines Prepare A Frightened Woman For Surgery, Help Her Recover From Anesthesia And Heal In Record Time.

She came in weeping, face drawn, obviously frightened. "I'm scheduled to have extensive periodontal surgery tomorrow," she said, "and I am panicked." She had been my patient since 2006 when she and her family lived in Houston. Subsequently, they moved to Scotland as her husband got transferred. No dentist in Scotland had been able to arrest her periodontal disease and, in a last ditch effort to resolve it, she came to Houston. I had known her as a strong, independent woman who could set goals and make them happen. She had been diagnosed with multiple sclerosis when she was fifteen and it was in remission. I had treated her successfully with *Phosphorus* for recurrent coughs and once for rectal bleeding. Later, she did well on *Ferrum phosphoricum.* When I saw her she was beside herself with fear. She was desperately worried the procedure might not be successful. In a week she and her sons were scheduled to fly to Angola to join her husband and she knew there would be no state of the art periodontists there. "I'm also worried about the sedation–that I won't wake up," she said. She was having diarrhea she was so scared. "I feel little," she said.

"What do you mean, 'little,'" I asked.

She held her thumb and forefinger slightly apart. "Little, like I'm little," she said. "I'm also angry at myself for being this way." In less than twenty-four hours she was to have a three to four hour surgery on her mouth and, in the state she was in, I wasn't at all sure she would go through with it so out of control was her anxiety.

I needed a medicine that had strong anticipatory anxiety plus one that covered diarrhea from being scared. I used the following rubrics in the repertory:

- Ailments from anticipation.
- Anxiety from anticipation.
- Fear of impending danger.
- Fear something will happen.
- Diarrhea from fright.

Gelsemium was the first choice. I remembered I had prescribed her *Gelsemium* for influenza that, after ten days, was still not clearing up. That was six months ago in January and *Gelsemium* had acted rapidly, restoring her to health overnight. Yes, I know. There is no connection between influenza and extreme anticipatory anxiety. But, in the world of homeopathy, where symptoms always trump logic, indeed, a connection is there. *Gelsemium* is, perhaps, the most famous medicine we have for influenza **and** it is one of the leading medicines for stage-fright and anxiety before major events such as examinations, operations, etc. In influenza, patients needing *Gelsemium* are usually dull, drowsy and often dizzy. They are apathetic and complain of general muscular weakness. A keynote symptom is that the body, including eyelids, feels heavy. She had been in that state in January. Now, however, she was showing the other side of *Gelsemium*, the one that panics before ordeals, imagined or actual. I gave her two doses plus sent her off with *Acetic acid* and told her to take the latter immediately on coming out of the periodontist's office. *Acetic acid*, prepared by diluting and succussing vinegar, is known to antidote the effects of anesthesia.

Two days after the surgery I saw her again. She seemed a different person. Her first words: "It brought all that emotion to a halt. There was a sense of, 'It's all right,' and I became calm. The crying stopped."

"How long did it take before you felt calm?"

"Within two hours."

I asked her to rate her anxiety before *Gelsemium* and right after. "Before it was 10/10. After it was 2/10." When I entered the periodontist's office the next morning, I was not looking forward to it, but I was composed. I no longer had that empty, clutched feeling in my stomach." I asked about how she did post-op. "I took the *Acetic acid* right away and I was definitely not groggy. When I had a colonoscopy in 2009, it was very different. I was way out. I don't remember leaving the office, getting in to a car, anything. After this surgery, I remembered everything."

For the swelling and pain she was feeling in the area operated on, I prescribed *Belladonna 10 M.* Within a day there was neither pain nor swelling.

A week post-op, she went to the same surgeon to have the stitches removed. Prior to the surgery, he had told her it would take four to six weeks to recover. When he looked, he was visibly surprised and said he had never seen such quick healing. "Your healing is a month ahead of schedule," he said.

Pre-op, post-op, homeopathy can make everything a whole lot easier. *Gelsemium* won't solve all pre-operation angst. And *Belladonna* won't solve all post-op pain and swelling. As always with homeopathy, the specific symptoms rule.

forty three

The Genius of the Provings

Practicing homeopathy is to marvel at the genius of Hahnemann who insisted that medicines be proved on healthy, intelligent human beings. Not on animals as do pharmaceutical companies when testing a new drug. Remember how miners used canaries? The pretty yellow birds are extraordinarily sensitive to toxic gases such as carbon monoxide and methane. A caged canary was taken into the mine. When the canary stopped singing, the miners bailed knowing the canary had died from toxic gases and that they'd be next. The pharmaceutical companies experiment on animals in much the same way miners used canaries—to learn when a new drug will kill the animal. Then they back the dosage off until they determine the "therapeutic dosage."

Using animals is a practice fraught with uncertainty as suggested by Dr. Arnold D. Welch, Department of Pharmacology, Yale University, who stated:

> In part because of possible major differences in responses to drugs in animals and man, the knowledge gained from studies in animals is often not pertinent to human beings, will almost certainly be inadequate, and may even be misleading.

[Taken from the Philip Morris 2001 stockholder meeting in which "PROPOSAL 4- Stop Funding Smoking Related Research Using Live Animals," was voted down by the Philip Morris Board of Directors.

Internet: http://www.gasp.org/pm2001prop.html]

Homeopaths know that giving a homeopathic medicine to healthy human beings is a far better way of understanding a medicine's effects than testing drugs on animals who, being without speech, cannot describe what they are undergoing. When a healthy man or woman takes a homeopathic medicine, they come under the sway of that medicine. The medicine acts on them and through them and they describe, in exquisite detail, all sorts of subtle physical sensations, strange pains and wonderful mood changes. As a result, our provings are filled with hundreds, sometimes thousands, of descriptive symptoms.

Because of provings, for the first time perhaps in the history of medicine, the **subjective** (what the patient experiences) and the **objective** (what the physician, and others, observe) are on an even footing. As a result, the physician is able:

- To understand disease from the viewpoint of the patient.
- To include all objective observations (physical examination, blood studies, x-rays, ultrasounds, scans, etc.).

JIVIN' CONNIE

Let's look at Connie, a bouncy woman with dazzling long blond hair. When I first took her case history in 1984 I was able to read most of her symptoms in the original proving of *Natrum muriaticum* by Hahnemann two hundred years earlier.

Always bubbly, always upbeat, she cut hair all day and entertained her clients non-stop with breezy banter, jokes clean or off-color, gossip, stories about the children, crime on the streets of Albuquerque, and so on. If you started a conversation she could run with it. And always music on the radio. Jivin' always jivin'.

And yet, when she came to my office, she was composed, even sedate, and almost introspective. "Yes, I'm always in a good mood—real mellow," she told me in 1984 when she was twenty-seven. "But it's a big front."

In that initial interview I learned she loved salt and starchy foods, couldn't stand oysters or jello (the texture) and was worse in the direct sun to the extent that she got a headache within minutes. It seemed clear she needed *Natrum muriaticum* so I asked a leading question: "If someone does you wrong, do you get even?"

Indeed, she did. "I once dumped a bag of sugar in the gas tank of a man who had messed with me. It ruined his engine."

Though she had had migraines since she was twelve, *Natrum muriaticum* took them away and they had never returned as of this writing in 2013. I was a beginning homeopath then and should have realized that *Natrum muriaticum* was her medicine, that it would have helped her in virtually all situations. I didn't and kept changing homeopathic medicines over the next twenty-five years. During that time, I watched as she developed breast cancer from which she recovered but continued to suffer arthritic pains and severe allergies. Then one day, I again spotted *Natrum muriaticum.* There is a proving symptom in *Chronic Diseases* [CD] by Hahnemann:

> Cheerful, merry and in good humor." [CD72]
> Very cheerful...she would have liked to dance and sing. –CD73.

Yes, this was Connie, my jivin' hairdresser. In fact, her passion, since childhood, had been dancing. Yet *Natrum muriaticum* also has the darker, introverted side, which she very much had, but rarely showed to the world. The person needing *Natrum muriaticum,* when in grief or sadness, prefers to deal with it alone. Grief she had had plenty of–a long series of painful, mostly failed, relationships with men.

I once asked her how she did with consolation. "When you're down and blue, do you like someone to be sweet to you, to console you?"

"Nah!" she shot back. "It looks weak." *Natrum muriaticum* is famous for rejecting consolation.

Most patients needing *Natrum muriaticum* show only the grief side, the sad side. They simply do not have the joyful, jivin' side. Because Connie almost exclusively showed the cheerful, upbeat side, I was constantly mislead (for twenty-five years!) and did not think of *Natrum muriaticum* until another homeopath made me aware of the rubric,

"Cheerful, with dancing, laughing and singing."

For the last three years, *Natrum muriaticum* has always helped her.

forty four

The Joy of Homeopathy

Homeopathy allows creativity. What do I mean, allows creativity?

The left brain permits logic, inference, deduction. It is the more scientific part. Chemistry and biochemistry have co-opted the left brain enabling more and more refined diagnoses. In the therapeutic realm, it has enabled the manipulation of molecules to create new pharmaceuticals.

The right brain permits feeling. It is the side that gives affective meaning, creates relationships, poetry, art, dance, and all that is alive and lively.

Man is the synthesis of the two sides. We have been created with two sides to our one brain. Conventional medicine glorifies the left brain. Homeopathy says, "Wait a minute. Your left brain is fine. It has brought order into medicine where there was none. It has allowed careful diagnosis and dazzling surgeries. But we also have this right brain. It must figure in medicine, too."

Homeopathy says, "Let's pay attention to the right brain as well as the left. Are not feeling states, subtle sensations–important, too?"

After all, homeopathic provings elicit all sorts of sensations, all sorts of feelings, as well as all sorts of functional changes–changes in thinking, changes in sleep, in digestion, in breathing, in the rhythm of the heart, constipation and diarrhea, all sorts of weird pains, dizziness, vertigo, incoordination, involuntary movements, etc. Homeopathy honors the right brain and says, "Let's hear from this side of you. It's important, too."

Creativity extends to case taking. The true homeopath aspires to empty his mind and make it completely receptive. He sees his mind as a blank canvas before a single brush stroke of paint has been applied. His mind is just there, waiting to receive. And then the patient speaks, gestures, moves this way and that and every word, every gesture, every movement is like a brush stroke painting a picture. The homeopath allows the patient to do the painting. He simply provides the canvas. He listens. He observes. His creativity is his receptivity. His mind is clean, open, waiting. The patient, using nothing more than his unique words and gestures, conveys an image, a unique image. Perhaps, the patient exudes a peculiar odor; perhaps the skin is discolored, has eruptions; perhaps his breathing is irregular; perhaps he is anxious, panicky, sad, overly lively or laughing uncontrollably; perhaps he lies, steals, cheats. If the interview takes place at the bedside, the homeopath notes how ruffled or neat the sheets are, whether there is a water jug on the table and how often the patient drinks, whether the patient is still or restless, sweating or feverish. Everything is taken into account—non-judgmentally.

From time to time, the homeopath may ask the patient to elaborate on something said; perhaps he may challenge the patient to be more exact, to go deeper. In the course of this most extraordinary interview, the image of the needed homeopathic medicine begins to come into view much as the artist's brush creates a picture.

By honoring the patient, by encouraging him to speak openly, honestly and fully about his problems, he allows the patient to create his own, vivid portrait of himself.

The homeopath brings out the artist in the patient by remaining quite still and receptive and allowing the drama that is the patient's life to unfold.

forty five

Allopathy and Homeopathy – Two Wings of One Bird

My intention in writing this book has been to explain homeopathic medicine–its philosophy and methodology–and to demonstrate how effective it can be especially in the treatment of chronic disease. Throughout I have shown bias in favor of homeopathy and against allopathy. But truth must go beyond bias. Allopathy's forte, as mentioned, is the use of chemistry and biochemistry allied with technology to diagnose disease with ever greater precision. Technological advances have permitted dazzling surgical procedures once unimaginable. Homeopathy's forte is in the treatment of chronic diseases not currently curable by conventional medicine.

Allopathy is thoroughly materialistic. Homeopathy is thoroughly vitalistic. They can and must be joined because man is both a material being and a vital being.

Osho, an Indian sage of the twentieth century, put it this way:

> "The whole of life consists of polarities: the positive
> and the negative, birth and death, man and woman,
> day and night, summer and winter. But these polar
> opposites are not only polar opposites, they are also
> complementaries. They are helping each other,
> they are supporting each other.
> "They are like the bricks of an arch. In an arch the
> bricks have to be arranged against each other. They
> appear to be against each other, but it is through their

opposition that the arch is built, remains standing. The strength of the arch is dependent on the polarity of the bricks arranged opposite each other."

Homeopaths must realize that technology is here to stay and will continue to advance. It is inevitable. The diagnostic capabilities made possible with technology are of benefit to all who practice medicine.

IF IT HAPPENS, IT MUST BE POSSIBLE

For over two centuries homeopathy has been repeatedly attacked as a spurious science, that it is nothing but placebo, and so on. Strangely, no physician who has seriously studied and practiced homeopathy has any doubts that homeopathic medicines indeed do work and are highly effective *when prescribed according to the Law of Similars.* When not so prescribed, indeed, they are no more effective than placebo.

As for the quack buster class with their frantic fictions that homeopathy can't work, therefore it doesn't work, they might listen to Richard A. Muller, professor of physics at the University of California. In an op-ed column in the New York Times, September 25, 2013, he wrote, "There is a theorem in science: if it happens, it must be possible."

Homeopathy has been happening all over the world for over two hundred years. Allopaths need to suspend judgment that homeopathy is nothing more than placebo. Believing homeopathy cannot work is nothing more than a belief and belief stifles inquiry. Science is not based on belief; it is based on open inquiry. The thousands of medical doctors, who have practiced homeopathy for the past two centuries and reported confirmed cures, were all schooled in scientific medicine (allopathy) firstly and left it for homeopathy because they found the allopathic model wanting, i.e., they were not getting people well.

Chronic disease is merciless and relentless, and to cure it requires the best of both schools of medicine. The medicine of the future will be an astute mélange using technology to diagnose and homeopathy to treat.

Acknowledgements

It is one thing to write a first book and quite another to get it published these days. This book was finished in June, 2012, and then gathered electronic dust as no publisher showed interest. If it were not for Melissa Patterson who read numerous books on self-publishing and then contacted the very helpful Travis Craine at CreateSpace and got the ball, i.e., me, rolling again, I doubt it would have ever seen the light of day.

My Albuquerque pal, Cortland Sutton, raconteur extraordinaire, former adman and English teacher, started urging me to write this book years ago. As I ploddingly wrote over many months, I would read chapter after chapter aloud and he would tell me which paragraphs and sentences "worked" and which did not. When I questioned him, he graciously explained why and ninety-five percent of the time he convinced me. His guidance and friendship were invaluable. Thanks to Elaine Muray of Albuquerque who did a meticulous job of final editing.

What abilities I have as a homeopathic physician are due, in some large part, to the numerous homeopathic doctors I have studied with over the years. Henry Williams, MD, and Maesimund Panos, MD, my first teachers, got me pointed in the right direction, i.e., following the precepts of the great Samuel Hahnemann and James Tyler Kent. Bill Gray, MD, spent a year studying with George Vithoulkas in Greece and then trained a small cadre of US homeopaths preparing us to work with Vithoulkas. His dedication and enthusiasm were wonderful. Time spent with George Vithoulkas, a Greek engineer turned homeopath, was exhilarating. George trained most of the leading homeopaths in Europe and the US during the 1970s and 1980s and I was fortunate to have studied with him. Francisco X. Eizayaga, the Argentine urologist turned homeopath, introduced me to his most useful ideas. Alfons Geukens, Belgian MD homeopath, was a great help as was the US naturopath, Paul Herscu, Rajan Sankaran of India, Andre Saine of Canada, Jan Scholten of Holland and Massimo Mangialavori of Italy. Other excellent teachers: Kim Elia and Will Taylor, M.D. both in the U.S. Tinus Smits, MD homeopath of Holland graciously asked me to edit his book, *Practical Materia Medica for the Consulting Room,* in the course of which I learned a great deal. Tinus was a special friend.

In recent years, I have made many journeys to Mumbai to sit with Dr. Prafull Vijayakar, one of the most talented homeopaths alive. My prescribing ability definitely increased after each visit. There have been many other fine teachers. We homeopaths are a small band of brothers and I am grateful to count myself part of this most unusual fraternity.

For over twelve years I have been teaching homeopathy in Latin America: in Cuba, Honduras, El Salvador and Guatemala. Having students means having to prepare and preparing means learning. My students, over the years, have become like family.

Of course, no book such as this one could be written without having consulted and treated thousands of patients. It is said your patients are your best teachers and it is certainly true. It is also said you learn from your mistakes and, certainly, my undeniable therapeutic failures led me relentlessly on studying, studying, studying, trying to master the elusive art and science of homeopathy. To learn even one homeopathic medicine well is a bit like living with someone for years. There is always yet another, fascinating new facet to be discovered. Each medicine is useful in acute and chronic illnesses, in infants, in children, in adolescents, in midlife and in old age. Each is useful in trivial complaints as well as life-threatening ones and everything in between. As we have hundreds of homeopathic medicines, the study of homeopathy is endless. Happily, practicing and teaching homeopathy is endlessly fulfilling.

Finally, I would like to acknowledge my great good fortune just to have been born, well-bred, decently educated, and lucky enough to have discovered homeopathy.

Karl Robinson
Albuquerque, New Mexico & Houston, Texas

Appendix to Chapter 2

MORE DETAILS ON HOW HOMEOPATHIC MEDICINES ARE MADE

There are two scales for diluting. One is the decimal scale, using the Roman Numeral 'x' signifying 10, the other is the centesimal scale, using the Roman numeral 'c' signifying 100.

- The decimal scale = one-tenth.
- The centesimal scale = one hundredth.

Using the decimal or 'x' scale one takes the mother tincture and puts one drop into a vial. Then **nine drops** of pure water are added. The vial is then capped or stoppered and the mixture is "succussed," shaken vigorously either by hand or by machine. At this point we have a one-tenth dilution. A drop of this solution is placed in a second vial and nine drops of water are added. Again, this mixture is succussed. We now have a one hundredth dilution (1/100). Done a third time, we have a one thousandth dilution (1/1,000), a fourth time a one ten-thousandth dilution (1/10,000), a fifth time a one-hundred thousandth dilution (1/100,000), and done a sixth time we have a solution containing one part in a million (1/1,000,000).

This procedure is known as a serial dilution. Each dilution is succussed. **Dilution + Succussion = Potentized substance**.

After 23 dilutions, using the decimal scale, it can be calculated that the solution contains no molecules. For those who remember chemistry, we have diluted beyond the negative of "Avogadro's Number" = 6.02 x 10-23.

Since it is awkward to use fractions with rapidly expanding denominators, we opt for 'x' meaning **one-tenth**.

- 1x = 1/10
- 3x = 1/000
- 6x = 1,000,000
- 12x = 1,000,000,000,000
- 30x = 1,000,000,000,000,000,000,000,000,000,000

When the centesimal or 'c' scale is used, instead of one-tenth, we now use **one-hundredth** so a 6c potentized substance is one that has been diluted using one part of the medicine to ninety-nine parts of water and then repeated six times. A 30c potency = the one to one hundred dilution has been carried out 30 times. A 200c = 200 dilutions. Some homeopathic medicines are diluted a thousand times and more. We refer to a one-thousandth potency as 1M and a one ten thousandth potency as 10M.

Why fractions become rapidly unwieldy.

- 1c = 1/100
- 6c = 1/000,000
- 12c = 1/000,000,000,000
- 30c = 1/000,000,000,000,000,000,000,000,000,000

Clearly, it is more convenient to write 30c rather than a fraction with 30 zeros.

- 200c = the denominator contains 200 zeros.
- 1M = a fraction with one thousand zeros in the denominator.
- 10M = ten thousand zeros.
- 50M = fifty thousand zeros.
- CM = one hundred thousand zeros.

The whole question of potency is an area where homeopaths differ, some favoring the lower potencies such as 6c or 12c repeated daily; others favor middle potencies such as 30c or 200c, others favor the higher potencies–1M, 10M, 50M, CM.

The middle and higher potencies are usually not repeated very often as most homeopaths adapt a wait-and-see attitude. The reason is that one homeopathic medicine, carefully selected, will often cause profound changes in the patient and repeating too often can be disruptive.

Most homeopaths will agree that the selection of the medicine is far more important than the potency.

Glossary

Acute illness – one of short duration ending either in death or recovery, e.g., a cold, bronchitis, pneumonia, meningitis, poison ivy, etc.

Aggravation – an intensification of the patient's symptoms that occur soon after taking the homeopathic medicine. Remember, homeopathic medicines cause the same symptoms they take away so the medicine, which mimics the disease, may briefly increase those symptoms. An aggravation can last from a few hours to several days and is a good sign suggesting the homeopathic medicine is acting.

Allopathy – a term adopted by homeopaths to refer to doctors of conventional medicine. "Allo-means other" and signifies the use of medicines that oppose or suppress the symptoms. A great many pharmaceuticals accordingly have, as a prefix, "anti-" as in anti-hypertensive, anti-depressant, anti-inflammatory, anti-convulsant, etc. Allopathy is the polar opposite to homeopathy (see homeopathy).

Characteristic symptom – any specific symptom or quality of the patient and/or the homeopathic medicine which stands out, e.g., diligence, laziness, constant lying, extreme honor, workaholic, strong willed, sentimental, meticulous attention to detail, extreme sensitivity to heat or cold, weather, unusual perspiration, food sensitivities, etc.

Chronic illness – any illness that persists over months and years and usually defies cure.

Common symptom – any symptom that is expected to accompany a complaint and that occurs so frequently that there is nothing unusual about it. Common symptoms are not used in homeopathic diagnosis as homeopathic prescriptions are mostly based on uncommon or **strange, rare** and **peculiar** symptoms (Chapter Four).

Concomitant – a symptom or condition that accompanies the principal problem. The two occurring together are out of the ordinary and can be helpful when deciding on the medicine (Chapters Thirty-two, Thirty-five).

Constitutional medicine – when a homeopathic medicine helps time and again a given individual we refer to it as his or her **constitutional** medicine. The term came into use after Hahnemann. The more correct term is **simillimum**.

Cure – the Holy Grail of **all** medicine and the most elusive. Certainly, more than the disappearance of symptoms or normalization of laboratory investigations. (See The Follow up, Chapter Forty)

Homeopathy – a system of healing that employs medicines administered in extreme microdosages that produce the same symptoms in healthy persons that they are intended to remove or cure in sick persons.

Isopathy – treating a condition, such as a poisoning, with a small dose of the **identical** substance, e.g., treating arsenic poisoning with homeopathic *Arsenicum album* or aluminum toxicity with homeopathic *Alumina* (Chapter Eight).

Keynote – a symptom which is strongly associated with a given homeopathic medicine, e.g., a strong interest in sex and a haughty manner are keynotes of *Platina.* Prescribing only on keynote symptoms can lead to wrong prescriptions. Better to use the **totality of symptoms**.

Law of Cure – when a patient has a truly curative reaction to a medicine, homeopathic or other, he or she is expected to improve:

1. From above downward.
2. From inside out.
3. In the reverse order in which symptoms originally occurred.

Law of Similars – central concept of homeopathic medicine that what a substance can cause (in healthy individuals) it can remove or take away or cure in a sick person. Often referred to as **Like cures like**.

Materia medica – descriptions of medicines, their sources, preparation and use. Most homeopathic materia medicas are composed of proving symptoms plus toxicological reports and some clinical reports. Some homeopaths have written their own material medicas with their own understanding of the homeopathic medicines. Hahnemann called his **Materia Medica Pura**.

Modality – anything that makes a symptom better or worse, e.g., sitting, standing, walking, pressure, heat, cold, wet, dry, etc. (Chapter Thirty-five)

Organon of Medicine – the original work by Samuel Hahnemann in which he expounded the principles and philosophy of homeopathic medicine. It is formatted in paragraphs, each paragraph numbered sequentially. Known informally as the "Organon," it is to this day studied and revered by homeopaths the world over.

Potentization – the preparation of homeopathic medicines by serial dilutions (one after the other) and succussions (see definition). All homeopathic medicines are potentized (Chapter Two).

Proving – a medical trial in which the homeopathic medicine is given to human subjects who are healthy until such time as symptoms are produced. The homeopathic medicine is then stopped. The symptoms often continue in the **prover** for several weeks. These are carefully recorded and later compiled into the **material medica** of that substance. Modern provings are double-blinded (Chapter Three).

Regular medicine also (**conventional medicine, scientific medicine, evidence based medicine**) – medicine as generally practiced by holders of a M.D. (doctorate of medicine) or D.O. (doctorate of osteopathy).

Repertory – a dictionary or compendium of symptoms (**rubrics**) used by homeopaths. All of the thousands of symptoms in a repertory are followed by one or more homeopathic medicines known to treat that symptom (Chapter Five).

Rubric – is simply a symptom but when the symptom appears in a repertory, it is known as a rubric.

Simillimum – the medicine most similar to the patient's symptoms. A true simillimum invariably acts curatively.

Similia similibus curentur (Latin) – "Let likes be treated by likes." A medicine known to produce symptoms in healthy individuals will remove those same symptoms when they occur in a sick individual. This phrase is the cornerstone of homeopathic philosophy.

Succussion – In the preparation of homeopathic medicines, after each dilution, the vial containing the medicine is vigorously shaken either by hand or machine. The person doing the succussion wraps his hand around the vial containing the dilution making a fist with the vial in the center. He then strikes that fist against a thick book or something similar. This thump appears to add energy to the diluted medicine (Chapter Two).

Susceptibility – people only fall sick when they are susceptible or vulnerable to a noxious stimulus. It could be a virus, bacteria, fungus, an allergen, a vaccination, an insecticide or pesticide, any sort of emotional shock, etc. Because we are all different, each of us is susceptible or sensitive to different stimuli. It is the degree of one's susceptibility that determines how well or poorly one can withstand noxious or harmful influences. For one person, a fifteen minute exposure to the summer sun causes a headache, for another, there is no reaction. One person gets diarrhea from half a glass of milk; another thrives on it. And so on.

Totality of the symptoms – a phrase coined by Hahnemann to refer to using all the symptoms of the patient (with special emphasis on the uncommon ones) to arrive at the most similar medicine.

Vital force – a term used by the founder of homeopathy, Dr. Samuel Hahnemann. It refers to an intangible energetic field that surrounds and penetrates the physical body. Homeopaths believe that in all illnesses the Vital Force becomes disordered producing symptoms. Homeopathic medicines, say homeopaths, balance or attune the Vital force which in turn causes the physical body to heal (Chapter One).

Made in the USA
San Bernardino, CA
13 October 2017